God's Technique to
Walk Run Relax

God's Technique to Walk Run Relax

Jack Nirenstein

iUniverse, Inc.

New York Lincoln Shanghai

God's Technique to Walk Run Relax

iUniverse books may be ordered through booksellers or by contacting:

iUniverse
2021 Pine Lake Road, Suite 100
Lincoln, NE 68512
www.iuniverse.com
1-800-Authors (1-800-288-4677)

ISBN-13: 978-0-595-40757-6 (pbk)
ISBN-13: 978-0-595-85121-8 (ebk)
ISBN-10: 0-595-40757-9 (pbk)
ISBN-10: 0-595-85121-5 (ebk)

Printed in the United States of America

Everything you should have learned before you ever started to train but didn't because you got the wrong instructions from coaches. The secret is out. There is only one possible way to run. Everyone does it marginally with bad form.

This book is dedicated to my daughter Debby, my son Michael, and my four grandchildren, Jeffrey, Richard, Morgan and Darcy.

Contents

Introduction

Revolutionary Revelation from God

I have been given the knowledge by our creator to change the face of health and fitness as the world knows it. I couldn't make such a seemingly outlandish statement if I wasn't certain I could convince you of the importance of the information I have received. Virtually every bit of God's whole system is unique in the health, sports, and fitness industry. How else but by a gift from God could someone like me, coming from an unrelated field, have envisioned what scientists, looking at the same evidence as I have, could not see?

People have always sought better ways to excel, but nobody has ever found the real power that makes you pick up speed. God has kept that knowledge a secret from everyone, even the professionals, until he showed the way to me. I feel blessed and humbled to be chosen to spread his word about the healthiest improvement technique that can transform you into a successful runner.

Rapid changes due to advances in science do not come easy. I found that I needed the help of God to overcome the industry's resistance to change. Books will need to be discarded. School coaches and professional trainers will need to be replaced. Qualified sports coaches will not be readily available to teach the real science. With the lack of a solid technique to improve runners, coaches rely mainly on outdated training methods and pressuring their athletes to perform. They attribute their failures to a perception that superior athletes can't be made, that they must be born with the talent.

However, everyone benefits from this technique by being able to move freely, speedily, and above all, healthily. Done God's way, running becomes by far the healthiest activity around. Circulation pumps blood from the feet and powerful legs upward throughout the body and pulls and returns the most blood to the heart.

You know that to be balanced for standing still your body needs to be centered over your feet. But nobody knew that you cannot stride ahead unless you switch your balance from being centered to being off-center. By removing your front support (lifting your toes or front foot), you start the secret process of being pulled forward by gravity. When walking, both feet are on the ground, but you lift the body with your back leg, taking the weight off the front foot. You then fall forward off the supporting foot behind you. You've seen pictures of runners in off-balance positions and probably did not notice that they are falling without pushing themselves. Those pictures show the runner's leg slanted behind his upper body's center (approximately navel high). It is important to note here that tilting the upper body does not shift your balance. You can stand still with a forward-tilted body and even run backward that way.

At this point you may find yourself confused. You just can't picture how to rebalance yourself for running. After all, your feet must keep landing in front of your upper body's center. That doesn't seem to be a forward shift of the upper body ahead of the foot. However, it actually is a forward shift, because the foot stays on the ground while the body's center moves farther ahead of the foot than when it landed behind the foot. That is the balance for holding a steady pace. A short slowdown and a long speedup keep you off balance for standing still but in balance for your speed.

One more thing needs to be clear so you can feel confidence in my proof. This has to do with how you reach your level pace. If you start off landing with your feet ahead of your body's center, as you do for a level pace, you will start running backward. This may sound strange, but you never start running by landing ahead of your body's center. To increase your speed with each step, your feet need to be landing behind your body's center. You do it that way but never noticed it. Notice your first three steps when going from a standstill into a run, and you will be surprised to see it happening. These revelations from God are the true science in that it cannot be and never was done another way.

With this knowledge you may think you're ready to start on your way to becoming a champion. Not so fast. There is more to learn. God gave you a sense of balance to protect you from exceeding your limits for being off balance without falling too low. That sense will tighten your muscles to hold you back. You need to be working with a lot more of his techniques before you can become efficient enough to compete.

God's Secret Way to Make a Baby Run

Looking back to the time when a baby learns to take its first steps, you can see a glimpse of God's secret running technique. The child falls uncontrollably forward, running into the mother's or father's arms before it is about to fall. The child later learns to bring its feet forward in time to correct its out-of-control running.

Now play that scenario in your head and look for the science God has revealed to me. It is the natural way a baby learns to fall forward into a run. The key is falling. Think about it: What makes you fall forward? You know the answer: gravity. Gravity is the power that takes the baby from a standing-still balance to an off-center running balance. If you are off center for standing still, you fall, catch, and lift yourself to keep moving forward. No one can see the outside power pulling people forward.

This information God gave me would allow anyone to become a champion. Ultimately, what you must do to win a race is to use my God-given technique in the forward reach of the feet: a landing spot, ahead of your upper body's center, that catches you but does not stop you. The farther off balance you can get yourself from a standing-still balance, the faster gravity will pull you. Therefore, you first drop your feet behind your body's center until you reach a faster pace than your competitors. Then, if you drop your feet with a shorter reach ahead, on average, than anyone else in the race, your level pace will win. That is the science given to me. Other methods cannot work.

Picking up your pace is easy when you have all the mechanics working well. All it takes is switching your landing spot from in front of your body to behind your body's center. You will pick up more speed with each step until you are ready to level the faster pace. To run at the faster level pace, you must keep yourself more off balance than at the slower pace. You do this by dropping your feet with a shorter forward reach ahead of your body's center.

Running through God's Universe

The direction in which you can move with speed changes with different forces of gravity. On a space station, your legs can only toss you head first with great speed. Try to walk forward, and you will find that you cannot. Your legs cannot push you forward anywhere in the universe. Lighter gravity on the moon than on Earth will not give you enough power to run as fast as you can on Earth. No power can come from your legs pushing the body forward. Your speed is only controlled by your off-balance position.

Running Techniques Compared
Speed process for every pace, from a walk to a sprint

TECHNIQUE	WHAT IT DOES FOR SPEED	CONCLUSION
Stride length and foot speed will increase your running speed.	It was never explained. Do the books want you to reach farther ahead to accelerate? Do they want you to exchange your feet faster? It won't work.	This is not a technique to increase speed. No amount of training with it will make you faster. A long reach ahead slows you.
Bringing your knees up high in front and your feet high in back will increase your running speed.	Swinging your body parts back and forth a long distance wastes time and energy. Gravity does not pull you forward during air time. It slows you down.	This is not a technique to increase speed. A sprint speed spreads the feet apart. It cuts off gravity's power to add more speed.

Running Techniques Compared
Speed process for every pace, from a walk to a sprint (Continued)

TECHNIQUE	WHAT IT DOES FOR SPEED	CONCLUSION
Tilting your upper body forward will increase your running speed.	It helps to start faster and safer on the first couple of strides. After that it is hard on the back muscles. You can stand still or even run backward with a forward-tilted upper body.	This is not a technique to increase speed. No amount of training with it will make you faster.
Pushing harder into the ground will increase your running speed.	Pushing harder tosses you higher into the air. Air time is slowdown time. Staying low shortens the stride for speed.	This is not a technique to increase speed. No amount of training with it will make you faster.
Dropping your feet directly under your body will increase your running speed.	You can only hop in place when you are in balance for standing still.	This is not a technique to increase speed. No amount of training with it will make you faster.
Dropping your feet behind your body's center of balance will increase your speed exponentially with each stride until your reach your pace.	Gravity pulls you faster with each step when you are off balance for holding a level pace by dropping your feet behind your center. When you reach your pace, a short reach ahead keeps you at a faster even pace than a longer reach will.	This technique is part of the discovery by Jack Nirenstein. Everyone runs this scientific way unconsciously. They cannot control their balance fully without more information from this book.

THE HEALTHIEST EXERCISE IS NIRENSTEIN'S RUNNING

ELEVATES:

• Relaxation	• Strength
• Circulation	• Manipulation
• Respiration	• Acceleration
• Joint Protection	• Neuromuscular Facilitation
• Speed	• Sports Performance
• Agility	

FITTER FITNESS FACILITATION

You can use all of your power and none of your resistance for relaxed power.

The strength and power you produce are diminished by the tension in your natural movement technique. As you may know, muscles can only shorten to move body parts in one direction. Muscles on one side of the body parts shorten to move those body parts in one direction. Muscles on the opposite side should be relaxed to let the movement happen freely. During any activity, more than half of your muscles need to be relaxed, so the muscles on the opposite side can move the body parts freely. With my self-transport technique (walking to sprinting); you will be able to do all your movements with relaxed muscles. You will not only be able to utilize more of your power, the technique will give you better circulation and respiration. It is impossible to derive much benefit from training when your technique is not perfected.

I have discovered that running at all speeds, from walking to sprinting, can only be done by using the power of gravity. This changes the old science of pushing yourself forward, which I show is wasted effort. The muscles across the front of the knee that absorb the landing and toss you up prevent the back muscles from moving the leg back. Your muscle power will make you jump higher on the moon than on Earth, but you won't be able to run as fast. Lighter gravity will not pull you forward as fast as heavier gravity will on Earth. When you are off balance for standing still, gravity will pull you to move. When you release your front support, you will always fall forward. During the running process, you stay off balance for standing still and in balance for your pace. You can't visualize this process because a lot more needs to be explained. However, here is a test you can do in one minute, including reading the instruction.

Let your body fall ahead of your feet or foot, and keep your feet dropping behind your body's center (navel high) for three or four strides. See yourself picking up speed with each step without pushing.

Explanation: What you did is the only way you can start and pick up speed with each step. You can't do it with a push. Tilting the upper body only helps you on the first step by making sure you don't use the back muscles and hurt yourself. It is also a faster way to shift your body ahead than from an upright position. After the start, staying low is useless and an unnecessary strain on the back muscles. You do not move forward by tilting your upper body; you can even run backward with a forward tilted upper body.

All this will be explained in greater detail, with pictures to help you visualize the technique better.

It's Not "Just Do It" Nonsense Anymore
It's Nirenstein's Running Just *Un*do It Science

Many can simulate the look of the movements of superathletes, but few are efficient enough to become that good. This is true with the vast majority of athletes, even the ones who train harder and longer than the superathletes. The Nirenstein technique for running can teach any-one to be even more efficient than the superathletes. If any of the superathletes were aware of the right technique, that person certainly would have written about it before me.

The fact that you can simulate the movements of superathletes and still be a mediocre runner, no matter how hard you train, indicates that you are doing some of it right but a lot wrong. Therefore, you need to learn what you are doing right and wrong and how you can perfect those movements for maximum results.

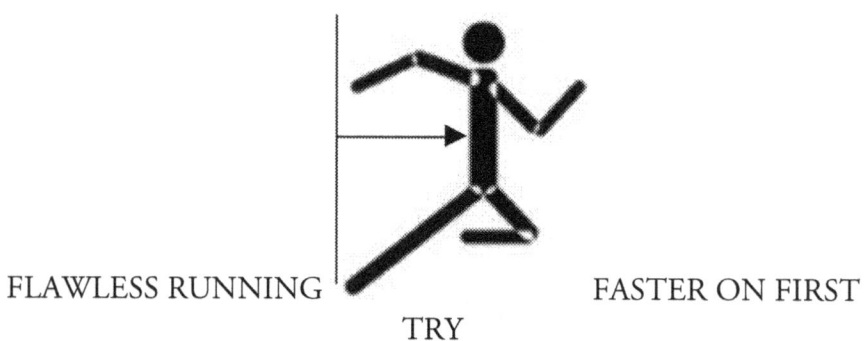

FLAWLESS RUNNING   FASTER ON FIRST
TRY
New healthy self-transport (walking to sprinting speeds)
eliminates tension, the biggest cause of illness.
Discovered by Jack Nirenstein

A preponderance of flaws in the way you move is causing unhealthy tension and jarring. Nobody knew, because it is a natural activity, that people have been doing it without instruction since they were infants. But scientists know that all movement has a mechanical efficiency. My discoveries are the first science of moving, with relaxation, at all speeds. Previously mysterious differences in technique are what made one run-ner better than another. Now no longer a mystery, it can be learned by everyone and used for relaxed speed or relaxed walking. You have the strength, but not the technique, to make you better right now. Train-ing, while running correctly, will make you stronger and faster than in your initial trial. Oscillating your legs and upper body parts rapidly takes a lot of time with practice. Consider how slow you are when you first learn to type, play a piano, or beat a drum. As with all coordination for speed, doing the activity you want to speed up and pushing the speed will make you stronger and more coordinated. Your muscles will recruit more fibers for strength and faster responsiveness. The neuromuscular facilitation and circulation will develop too.

Everyone runs my way but adds tension by resisting the movement when trying to push. The pushing muscles—gluteus and hamstrings—can't move you about, because the opposite muscles—quadriceps and calf muscles—that absorb the landing and lift you up won't let you push. The legs are positioned under your body for tossing you straight up, head first. If you are not falling first, the legs will not take you forward.

Everyone lands off balance for standing still and in balance for moving. Being off-balance for standing still causes you to fall forward for the purpose of moving. The image above shows that the runner is off balance for standing still and is falling forward. You should be able to see that gravity pulls you forward when your leg is slanted behind your body. My techniques will get you to release opposing muscles, which is the only way to relieve tension.

Think about this principle: The more you do of the wrong thing, the slower you run. When you are told to increase your stride, just a little for speed, you will actually slow down. The more you increase your reach ahead, the more you slow down. Your upper body twist is used only to shorten the stride. A shorter reach ahead allows you to set yourself more off balance and run faster. The speed increases your stride while you are trying to keep it short so that you can exchange your feet faster. It is harder work to push for greater speed than it is to stay at your level. If you want to get faster, you need to do more hard work than your body is currently accustomed to doing. Your heart and breathing muscles get stronger too. Pretty soon speed becomes easier.

Today's training methods have little chance of success, because nobody knew the mechanics to use for speed before me. Obviously, if your mechanics aren't producing speed, working harder will make you tense, slow you down, and cause injuries.

Don't expect any of the magazines to publish an article on these techniques. If the knowledge becomes widespread, the entire fitness industry will experience a total upheaval. Training camps and publications will be obsolete. Many fitness authorities agree with my technique but still stay with their techniques that are diametrically opposed to the physical laws.

Biomechanics Can't Make You Run: It Acts Only as the Reactive Force to Gravity

Gravity pulls you forward when your leg is slanted behind your vertical body. You can see what you and everyone else missed when you look at the previous image of a runner. The slanted leg is acting like a slanted pole; the runner will fall forward when the weight is not centered over the base. The foot stays in place and rolls with gravity, pulling the top of the leg forward. This was always in plain view but not picked up as a true science for running. Where does this knowledge help us to run? Nowhere yet with only this bit of information.

Now I feel comfortable in telling you that I invented the full physical method to become a champion and even break records. I think you can see something enlightening here and will give me a chance to prove I am not delusional about my mechanics for running. By the way, I combine all the speeds, from a slow walk to a sprint, as one process. When you see how gravity works in this process, you can see why. It will enhance your life by making it healthier and relaxed, with an improvement in performance in the most used activity, self-transport.

In the past twenty years I have written three books and produced a video. I have given lectures and been interviewed by local TV, radio, and newspapers. I also coached a high school runner with spectacular results. At seventy-seven years old, I have run seven marathons and won mile and hundred-meter events. I am presently a fast sprinter for any age.

For TV and lectures, I demonstrate my technique using members of the audience or myself. It is just as convincing as using a champion. I have the person stand with one foot in front of the other, lift the front foot, and show the person falling forward. Then I have the person lift the back foot and show the person falling backward. I can use other simple demonstrations to show other aspects of my technique. My technique can be shown as hard science by demonstrating how the angle of the leg at foot strike determines the pace for everyone alike. Simple proof is to have you run very slowly and abruptly pick up to a very fast pace. You will notice that you must change the angle of your foot strike to behind your body's center to pick up speed with each step. I can also demonstrate how every other technique is not only dangerous but also cannot make you run. If you are pushing instead of falling, you won't be able to get started with your first stride.

Everyone runs with gravity, but they run recklessly and inefficiently. They do all sports movements with limited effectiveness and lose a lot of power due to a lack of technical knowledge.

Technique Is First
Training Is Last

The world desperately wants to learn what champions know. People have been reading their books, watching their videos, and attending their camps to find out. What runners learned from champions is the standard key to running technique: stride length and foot speed. They want you to get stronger to stride longer and exchange your feet faster. The instructions they are giving runners is not at all what they did to become champions. It is not because they don't want to let their secret be known, but because they don't know what they were doing to be fast. The technique they teach is opposite to what they actually did. Here's why: You can stride much longer than a sprinter right now, but you won't be able to go any faster than a slow walk with your longest stride. You can also exchange your feet faster than a sprinter with a very slow and short stride.

What the champions know is all wrong. That is why so few of the good athletic prospects they train ever reach anywhere near their potential. This observation can now be made, because I have discovered the real key to running. Here it is: falling speed, lifting speed, and twisting speed. Everyone runs this way because nothing else will make you run. Striking the ground with an extremely slanted leg will make you fall forward fast. Lifting quickly while falling fast changes the forward fall to a parallel direction with the ground before you fall too low. The shoulders and feet twist fast in opposite directions to return the foot more quickly for the next stride in order to catch you before you fall. The Nirenstein running key is just an outline of a small part of the process. It is not detailed enough to make it work for you. The key is one of many things you need to do better before you can perform well and avoid injuries.

You do many things wrong that crush your joints, grip your muscles, and cut your circulation. The Nirenstein full key goes beyond the basic key to correct all your faults. They are all hard science that replaces the old way.

 Only the front muscles work across the knee.

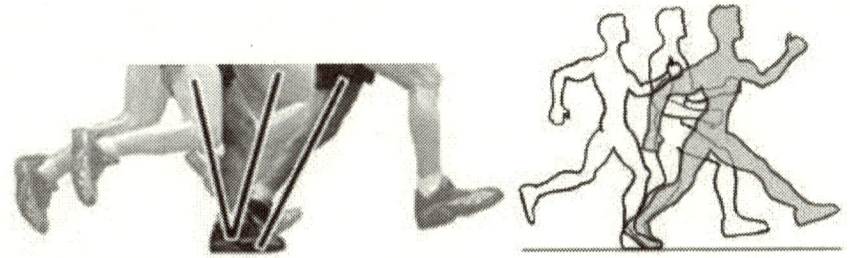

A slanted leg falls forward while rolling on the foot.

The back muscles of the leg should be relaxed; because they cannot do any work other than hold the upper body to prevent it from lurching forward at landing. The front muscles of the leg lock the knee to prevent collapsing and toss the body up. They prevent the back muscles from pulling back to push you forward. Falling is the only thing you are able to do to move forward.

The leg acts like a pole. It is locked at the knee joint, so it can't bend. It vaults the body forward the way a vaulting pole would. It does this by falling forward from a pull by gravity.

Now you can see what you missed seeing about how you run. Researchers, champion runners, and champion coaches missed seeing it as well.

Scientists know that all movement has an ultimate specific technique that will take athletes to their highest level of performance. It is accomplished by making the movement totally efficient.

They also know that all the searching has never produced that ultimate technique. Some scientists have come up with theories, but none has lived up to its hype.

Here is how falling gets you to pick up speed with each step until you reach your even pace: The striking point where the foot strikes the ground sets the speed. To pick up speed with each step, you must strike the ground behind the body's center and keep it striking there until you reach your level pace. A slow runner drops the feet behind the body's center for a few steps and levels off by reaching ahead. A fast runner keeps the feet dropping behind the body's center for more steps to reach a faster pace.

Here is how falling keeps you at a level pace: When you reach your level pace after having taken the amount of steps with the foot striking the ground behind the body's center, you then change the striking point. To even the pace, you start striking the ground ahead of the body's center. A faster runner strikes the ground a shorter distance ahead of the body's center than a slower runner. What keeps you falling when at an even pace striking the foot ahead of the body's center? Take note: The reach ahead of the body's center is shorter than the length the foot rolls behind the body's center. That keeps you off balance for standing still and at your level pace.

The more you do of the right technique (Nirenstein's) for speed, the faster you will run. The more you do of the champion's technique (stride length and foot speed), the slower you will run. Champions do it the Nirenstein way of reaching short but have the illusion that they are reaching far ahead. Try it both ways to compare. Reach as far ahead as you can (champions' way), and you will find that you slow down to a slow walking pace. Reach behind your body as far as you can (Nirenstein's way,), and you will pick up the most speed you are able to reach. This proves the Nirenstein technique is the new science. The runner who drops his feet more to the rear than the other runners always wins the race. It can't be done another way.

I have to rely on people to evaluate the technique for themselves. There are no experts on running technique other than myself.

Running technique is a vital prerequisite to training.

Don't Train without Your Brain

In outer space, you can jump head first and fly forever, but you can't fall forward to walk or run. On the moon, you can jump higher than you can on Earth, but you can't run as fast. Heavier gravity pushes you faster than lighter gravity.

The government agencies that deal with health and exercise should look into testing this. However, they won't. The President's Council on Physical Fitness and Sports is made up of top experts. They would not like to lose their status as experts to a lone infidel with the correct technique. They will respond to anyone else they can impress. Schools at every level will be vulnerable for lawsuits if they are teaching the wrong technique. When you try to do what's good, you might have to hurt a lot of people in the process.

How to Drop Your Feet to the Rear to Start Speeding Up Exponentially to Your Level Pace

When people hear about moving by gravity, the top question they ask is "how do I drop my feet to the rear?" This query shows that people don't know what they are doing to make themselves run. They are surprised when I tell them that they already do it when they run, that nobody can run without doing it.

To notice how you always start out to run, do it for three or four strides. Notice that you naturally use God's method to go from a standstill to a fast pace. Keeping your body low and knees bent keeps you safe at the start. Notice when you take those few steps to increase speed that your feet automatically drop behind your body's center (approximately navel high). Getting faster at manipulation of your entire body will allow you to drop your feet farther back and do it for more steps. That is the way a sprinter does it also, without knowing it. Being aware of the need to be more off balance for speed allows you to develop your oscillations to exchange your feet fast. Your sense of balance tries to keep you from falling, so it will tie up your muscles if you are falling too low.

The speedup phase starts the forward movement. What follows is the level pace where the feet slow the body down slightly by striking the ground ahead of the body. A faster even pace is accomplished with a short reach ahead for the foot-strike. The slowdown and speedup is part of a level pace.

The movement starts with the supporting leg slanted behind the body's center of balance. The top of the leg topples forward first, and then the lift raises the body while moving forward. This keeps the body moving parallel to the ground. The raised leg comes forward and drops with a forward reach that will keep you off balance for standing still and in balance for maintaining your pace.

Seeing the big picture: Gravity makes you fall forward and down; the lift keeps you moving parallel to the ground.

How a Sprinter Uses Gravity

Figures A to D show one leg going through a complete cycle. At right, figures A to C show the other leg.

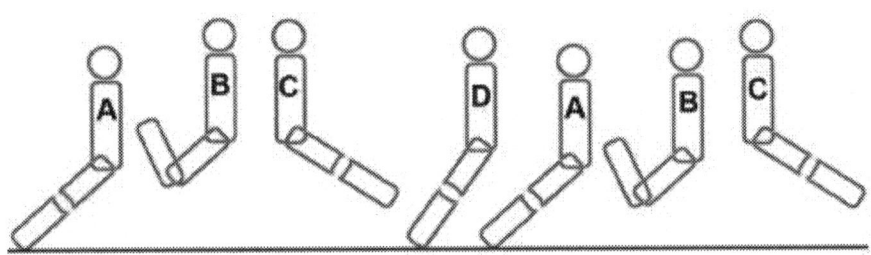

A sprinter takes approximately twenty strides, with each stride being exponentially faster than the previous one. The foot strikes down as far as possible behind the body's center of balance to get the strongest pull from gravity. The phase shown here is the speedup sequence when the sprinter reached maximum speed and is about to level the pace. When the sprinter levels the pace, the foot will strike down at the shortest reach ahead of the body's center of balance that the sprinter can make it in order to keep the pace fast.

A. The foot is dragged back by the ground, while the body is pulled forward by gravity. This happens with great speed, so the leg can't be stopped from reaching high in back.

B. Momentum sends the foot very high before the sprinter can start to swing the leg forward.

C. The foot is swung forward as fast as the sprinter can do it, so the foot overstrides in the air.

D. The foot is dropped back and down, while the body zooms past the foot. The foot strikes down as far behind the body's center of balance as the sprinter can make it.

A., B., C.: The other foot goes through the same cycle. The foot is dragged far back, and the body is pulled forward very fast. The next stride begins with the same cycle until you get to maximum speed. When that is achieved, the foot reaches ahead of the body's center. The forward reach is kept as short as possible. You should never try to increase the spread of the feet. The spread is an unavoidable inefficiency and slows you down.

Walkers, joggers, and runners do the same thing as a sprinter to pick up speed. They do it for less strides and pick up less speed. They do not need to exert themselves as much to try to shorten their stride length. A medium stride length is more comfortable for walking, jogging, and running.

Foreword

Movement comes naturally to people from the time they are born. A self-learning process starts early on to turn clumsy, stiff action into smoother, coordinated actions for various endeavors.

Many runners try to use their natural talent with rigorous training and wonder why they still can't reach anywhere near the level of performance that a few others do. They turn to coaches to improve their running performance, as do athletes in all other sports. They look to go beyond what they are able to achieve on their own trial and error attempts.

If you've been disappointed in the past by false claims, you must see what I do. I start out on the very first page with my initial discovery and prove that none of the coaches were able to teach you how to run. They couldn't because they learned it wrong in school.

Too many athletes are underachievers because the information that is passed on to them about form is actually making them worse than they might have been on their own.

So that I can have the opportunity to help you, I am obligated to warn you of the dangers you could be heading into by getting wrong form advice. If you can't run properly, you certainly won't get the benefits from training programs promising to make you faster.

In addition to the detrimental advice you get from other sources, the rest of what they teach is meaningless instruction. They tell you to run softly, lean, push off your toes, have good posture, breathe deeply, and relax. That isn't what an instructor should be teaching. As instructors, they should tell you how and why it should be done a certain way. That is what I do, because I know how and why.

I can tell you that my techniques are the right ones because they are different, and they improve you on the first try. Tell my technique to the highest authorities and see if they will dare to reply. They don't with me.

The Diametrically Opposed: Standard Science and the Nirenstein Running Method Compared

The standard running method uses a *backward* push by the leg for lengthening the stride to increase speed.

The basic Nirenstein method uses a *forward* push by the leg to raise the body as it falls to the ground. The stride is kept comfortably short. Foot placement controls speed.

The standard method drops the body to the ground by forcing the leg back and up while the foot is on the ground. When the supporting leg moves behind the body, it can only swing up. Everyone presses down and forward to raise the body, while hopelessly trying to push back and up.

The Nirenstein method lifts the body to keep it level with the ground by pressing down and forward. The front muscles are used to lift by pressing down and forward.

The standard method allows gravity to drop the body straight down by releasing the support muscles.

The Nirenstein method uses gravity to make you fall forward to run. You stand neutral on the ground and roll on the foot.

The standard method can never be used by anyone because it is impossible for the leg to support the body when it is pushing back. Pushing back is not a viable method.

The Nirenstein method is used by everyone because gravity is the only force used to run.

The standard method uses science that can't be applied to running.

The Nirenstein method of using gravity to make you fall forward when you are not balanced is easy to understand.

The standard method will not make you run faster on the moon, where the muscles can move the body more easily because of lighter gravity—this is proof that a push doesn't work.

The Nirenstein method makes you run faster on earth than on the moon because you can get a harder push from gravity.

The standard method has no additional features because you can't even get started to run.

The Nirenstein basic method accompanies a complete course that adds improvement after improvement. Each technique will improve your form on the first try. Academic credentials would not have taken Nirenstein in the right direction. His method is unique in the industry. He developed it over many years. This is his third book on running technique. There is only one way possible to run, so everyone does it without knowing that gravity is the initiating power. Nirenstein has the only technique for running.

Nirenstein isn't looking to hurt the industry. He has been informing the leaders about his technique, but they choose to look the other way.

**Muscle Control
Just Undo It**

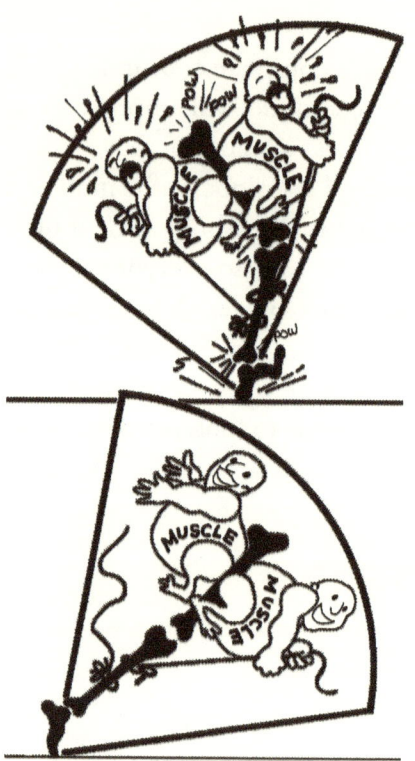

There has never been a known method that would allow you to relax the muscles that oppose your movements. But now a method has been found that will allow you to do just that, and now it can be learned, and it's simple. This method not only gives you freedom of movement, it also opens up your circulation channels as well.

You can prevent and relieve cramping by using this method. Muscles can only pull to move the skeleton by shortening themselves. They can't push by lengthening themselves. One side of a joint does the pulling while the opposite side is supposed to totally relax. But no muscles relax when you don't know technique. It never happens by just doing it.

Tension from poor muscle control compress the chest and can be life-threatening in the worst-case scenario, and otherwise unhealthy. Performance is also diminished when muscles are out of control. Combining my relaxation control method with my running biomechanics techniques will do wonders to help you achieve your goals.

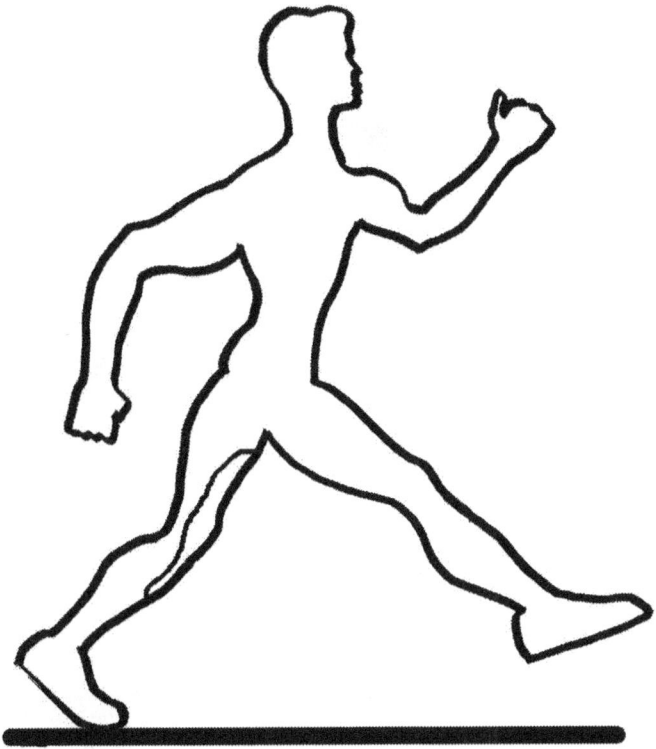

Quadriceps muscles push the leg down and forward to toss the body up. The leg can never push back at the same time, no matter how hard you try to do it.

The foot is also pushed down and forward while the body is moving. The foot is rolling along with the body, being pulled by gravity. When the body is ahead of the foot, it will always fall forward without a push.

This is not the complete explanation of how the running movement takes place, and it is the same for everyone. So read on and get it all. How you should move every part of your body becomes obvious with simple science when I point out all the things that were missed by others.

The Blind Leading the Blind

Take a look at the natural running picture below, and I will show you something that nobody else has been able to see before. Notice that the runner cannot stand still in this position. He has been falling forward and then jumping up while he is falling. Gravity was pulling his body straight down, but his leg won't let his body go straight down, so it vaults him down and forward. The jump keeps him from falling and sends his body moving level with the ground. This is obvious proof that gravity pulls you forward. It doesn't have to be tested because everyone already knows that any object that isn't centered on its base is going to fall in the direction the weight is positioned. While gravity running is not a new concept, my method is the first and only way to make it work.

Another fact worth noting is that you cannot shift your weight ahead of the foot with a push by muscles. From a standstill position, as well as in a running motion, you need to position the foot to the rear of the body to let gravity shift your weight. The foot rolls on the ground like the bottom of a vaulting pole.

These introductions to my unique techniques are but an infinitesimal part of the vital information you should learn before you run again.

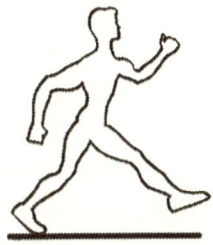

"Running—Just Undo It" Is the Symbol for a New Science

In the past, there has been a dismal lack of intelligence about the biomechanics of running. Everyone runs correctly, but they often let bad science interfere. Natural inclinations and the methods prescribed in professional running circles lead runners to bad mechanics. Anyone who says that it is best to just run your natural way shows a gross oversight of the poor methods that affect form and the way runners underperform when they run. The standard science of pushing hard for a longer stride sounds logical, but you will see that it actually opposes the action. You accept it without thinking about the obvious. The longer you make the stride, the slower you are able to run. More surprising but equally obvious is the fact that you can't push back to the ground when you are running. If you are not falling forward, you will not be moving forward—no matter how hard you attempt to push. The force of gravity, rather than muscular force, makes you fall.

After you learn my new science I will give a step-by-step way to use my method. This new science will convert the skeptics who find it hard to believe that running is a technique-intensive activity.

Recognized leaders in the science research and science development fields of running should never have been taken seriously. They have all failed to solve the mechanics of what it takes to run. My techniques are not only better; they are the *only* way to run effectively. They will help you achieve better health, safety, and performance when compared with running the old way.

Some people think it is bad taste to be critical of other authors who have written books on running. I feel that by comparing my books with theirs, I will steer people away from other bad influences. Many other books have flaws in biomechanics that can cause injury to runners, so I must explain why standard running books are wrong in order to convince them. It is hard enough to convince someone that great running can be learned after they have heard from the experts that it can't be. Colleges and coaches teach the same. Running camps being at the forefront of coaching is a good place for me to challenge the professional field; hence my attack on the proverbial "Just Be Natural" slogan. Professionals teach runners to push themselves forward for a longer stride to increase speed. I prove that it is impossible to push back at the ground while you are pushing down and forward to jump with your quads. I also prove that only gravity can push you forward to run.

I am not the first person to say that gravity pushes you forward to run. However, I am the first person to figure out the biomechanics to get the right effects from using gravity to run.

People do not understand the biomechanics they are using when they run. They can be instructed by coaches to do impossible gyrations, and they are convinced they are actually doing the impossible when, in truth, they are not. It is equally important that I point out the prevalent method of running to make a comparison between the good and bad ways to run. If you don't know any better, you will follow the wrong advice and wind up on the injured list.

Falling First, Then Jumping, Is the Basic Power to Move from One Spot to Another in Walking and Running Activities.

You cannot jump from one spot to another without falling first. Only gravity can shift your weight away from a standing, motionless position. On a space station you can jump up and go up forever, but you can't shift your weight forward to walk or run. On the moon you can't run as fast as you can on earth. Less gravity will allow you to jump higher, but it won't pull you as hard to move forward. After you take your first step, momentum and gravity keep you moving the rest of the way.

There are two different ways to take your first step. The first way begins when you are standing with your feet together and your weight is centered between your heels and toes. You need to position your feet to be off center. To do that, lift your toes, and your weight will be ahead of your heels, which is now off center, and you will fall forward. The second way is to stand with one foot in front of the other. Your weight is centered between both feet. Push up with the back foot, and your weight will be only on your back foot, so gravity will send you ahead of the front foot and the process of walking or running begins.

After the first step, the length of the reach of the foot ahead of the weight controls the pace. A shorter step in front of the body creates a faster pace by lessening the slowdown section. Each stride has a slowdown and a speedup section during the support phase, when the foot is on the ground. The foot lands in front of the body and lifts off the ground behind the body.

Hitting the Particular Landing Spot ahead of Your Body Is the Only Way to Control Your Pace.
It Is Similar to Placing a Vaulting Pole in Position for a Low Horizontal Vault.

There are a slowdown section and a pickup section during the support phase in the vault of the leg. Planting your foot ahead of your body starts your body moving from behind your foot to a point directly in front of it. This is the slowdown phase of the vault. When the moving body position is directly over the foot, the pickup phase begins and lasts until the foot leaves the ground behind the body. The slowdown and pickup combination during the support phase keeps you at a steady pace. You cannot see the precise placement of your leg, but that won't affect your ability to control your speed. You can feel yourself dropping your feet back toward the vertical position of the leg for a faster pace.

Landing with your foot directly centered under your body can only be done in a vertical hop. There is no other way to shift your weight than by dropping your feet off center.

At a sprinting speed, the foot lands close to the center of the body for a shorter slowdown phase and a longer pickup phase. The faster the flight of the body, the faster the foot gets flipped back by the drag of the ground moving away faster.

At a medium speed, the foot drops farther ahead of the center of the body than at a sprint. The slower drag from the ground doesn't flip the leg as high.

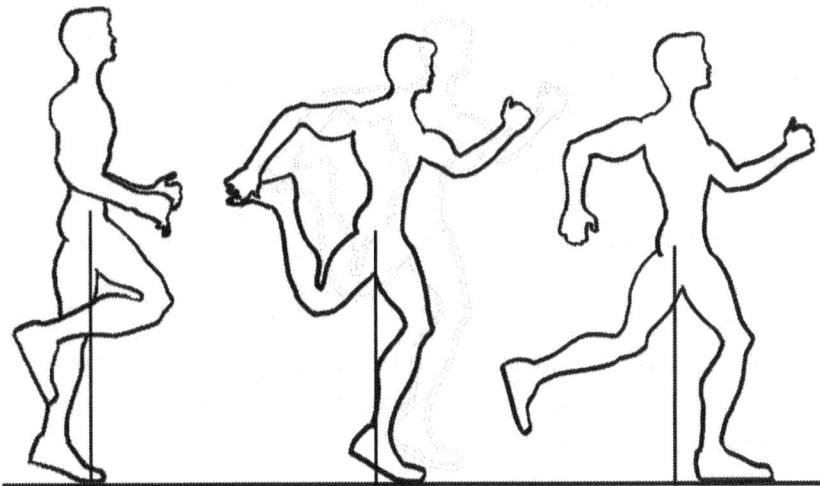

Other Techniques to Run with Gravity Don't Work

Some people heard about a method of using gravity to run and told me that someone else had the same method as mine. That method is completely different than mine. The other method is controversial; mine is a hot potato that professionals hope will never become widespread information. The following information measures my method against the flawed gravity method.

Flawed: When running, lean forward to the point that you are falling forward.

Undo It: Tilting your upper body does not affect speed. There are champions who break records with an upright body. You can stand still with your body tilted way forward, and you can even run backward with a forward body tilt. Gravity is the only force that can shift your weight ahead of your foot, so *you* can't shift your weight to let gravity pull you forward as you were told to do in the flawed method.

Flawed: Land with your feet directly under your body.

Undo It: Landing with your feet directly under your body's center of gravity will not allow gravity to push you forward. You cannot fall forward from a centered stance. When you jump from a centered stance, you can only go straight up. Your body cannot be shifted ahead from a vertical position by pushing it. Your foot needs to do the shifting by landing to the rear of your body's center, or else you will be staying in place. If you are hopping in place, only dropping your feet to the rear of your center will send you forward. To fall forward, you must be falling before jumping. Changing your landing position alters your speed. After you land, you cannot shift your body forward. Gravity does it all for you from that point on. Consider the extremes to better understand what I am saying: If you land with your feet extended as far ahead of your body as you can, you are running as slow as possible for your body. On the other hand, if you land with your feet as far behind you as you can, you will be running as fast as possible for your body. This is absolute proof that your landing spot—in relation to your center of gravity—determines your pace. Your exact position is not noticeable, but you will see by my method that you don't need to know where it is; you can feel it by a method that I describe later in this book. You cannot maintain an erect position by keeping a straight line from head to toe while running. The legs rotate forward and back at the hip, so your body varies its position. This variation is a vaulting rotation not mentioned by other methods. See later on in this book for an explanation.

Flawed: Land and stand with your knees slightly bent at all times.

Undo It: You cannot run with your leg evenly bent at the knee at all times, or you will fall. Your knee and your ankle work together to extend your leg, in order to raise you from the forward fall and keep you level with the ground.

Flawed: After your foot hits the ground, pull your foot straight up to your butt using your hamstrings.

Undo It: Lifting your feet should only be done slightly in a walk and slow jog. The faster you go, the higher your feet are flipped in a circle around the knee as the axis. After your foot leaves the ground, your knee continues behind the body—not forward—to bring your foot straight up. Your knee comes forward after having traveled back first. Your foot also travels back before being brought forward to land ahead of your body. You should not assist the natural flip of your foot in a faster run. You cannot bring your feet straight up in a run. The speed of your upper body matches the speed of your foot being dragged backward and flips your foot back off the ground. The other gravity methods state that you should exchange your feet fast, but they tell you to lift your feet for a longer travel away from the ground and a longer travel back. But it doesn't make sense to travel a longer distance and get there faster than you can by using a shorter distance.

Flawed: Pushing yourself forward against gravity is too hard.

Undo It: Pushing yourself forward is not too hard *because* it works against gravity; pushing is impossible to do at all. You are jumping while spinning forward in a fall. It is common knowledge that your knee rotates forward for a jump. The forward rotation by your quadriceps pushes your foot down and forward, so you can't use your hamstrings or hip extender muscles to push backward. When you try to push back, the tightening of your whole leg from opposite sides pits the hamstrings against the quadriceps, and does not allow your foot to push back. It is attempted, but never accomplished.

Flawed: Land on your toe.

Undo It: Landing on your toe is not a particular method or innovation as it may seem. Many runners resort to it for less impact to their joints. The toe landing is well-known for being much easier on your joints, so this "method" doesn't need to be tested. It lessens the impact on your joints the first time you try it. Toe landing does not affect your potential for speed in anything but a sprint. In a sprint, you must get off the ground before you drop too low. By rolling on the toe, you cut off the excessive backward travel of your foot. The only way you can get off the ground is from your toe. By starting out on your toe, you can get off the ground in time to avoid the excessive lowering of your body. Landing on your toe during a sprint—with your heel low to the ground—allows you to lift up with your toe together with your knee. The lift enacted while you are falling keeps you level with the ground.

Landing on your toe causes unnecessary problems for distance running. Your calves and Achilles tendons are endangered by the severe leverage applied against them. Your foot is at a right angle to the leg, so the leverage is great. There are eight things you can do to lessen the impact and make a flat landing eight times softer than the way runners ordinarily land flat. See them in Chapter 16.

My first running book was not a takeoff on another method of gravity; it was published many years prior to the other more recently published book and video.

I can say without fear of contradiction that any biomechanics scientist cannot dispute my method of biomechanics for running. As a matter of fact, testing it is redundant because it works the first time and every time thereafter. Saying that it must be tested is like saying that "jumping in a lake will get you wet" needs to be tested to see if it is true. So when you hear people say that my method needs to be tested, tell them to jump in a lake.

Virtually all runners will be injured by using their natural style or the dangerous advice given by professionals. The following is some of the mistaken advice on running given by other professionals.

The Standard Academic
Techniques Coaches Learned
Are Wrong

Their Advice: Push harder against the ground to increase speed.

My Response: You are just pushing against your leg that is pushing forward to jump. Experts know that to jump you use your front muscles across the front of your knee to rotate the joint forward. It is only an illusion when you feel that you can rotate your knee joint backward to push and forward to jump. It may feel like you are doing it, but it will never happen.

Their Advice: Push off from your toes.

My Response: This advice is funny. Have you ever seen anyone push off from his or her heels? This advice seems to imply that the harder you push off from your toes, the faster you will be running. This is not correct. The harder you push off from your toes, the higher you jump; the more time spent in the air, the more you over-stride and slow down.

Their Advice: Land with your feet directly under your body in a pose fashion, then shift your weight and gravity will push you forward.

My Response: If you land with your feet directly under your body, you will be running in place (actually hopping in place). When you run at an even pace, your feet *must* drop ahead of your body. It is impossible for runners to drop their feet under their body and walk or run. To run, gravity shifts your weight ahead of your foot to fall forward while you are jumping. The incorrect advice instructs you to shift your weight ahead without gravity. If you could shift your weight ahead, then it's too late for gravity to work. Besides, your landing spot changes to increase or decrease speed. The more you drop your feet toward the rear, the faster you run, and vice versa.

Their Advice: Lengthen your stride to increase speed.

My Response: Your stride is forced to lengthen when you increase speed. For every increase in body speed, there is an opposite increase in the speed of the ground pulling the foot back. The increased speed of your grounded foot flips the leg farther back and up. This extra length in the stride would slow you down if you didn't increase the speed of your returning foot. The more you try to shorten your stride, the faster you can run.

Their Advice: Lean for speed.

My Response: Slanting your upper body does nothing to shift your weight to make you fall. You can slant your upper body forward and stand still—or even run backward. Fast running can be done equally as well with an upright body as it can with a tilted one. Learning to shift your weight using either way will make you run faster.

Their Advice: Turn your hip to push your foot forward fast.

My Response: Turning your hip turns your foot sideways. Hitting the ground that way will twist your joints and injure you.

Their Advice: Bring into play the muscles in the buttock and back of your thigh to push you forward during the support phase. By doing this you will run faster.

MY RESPONSE: The muscles of the buttock and back of the thigh are only used to prevent your upper body from lurching forward at landing. The landing starts with a slowdown phase, and your body wants to continue flying fast. Your back muscles cannot push you forward because your muscles on the front of your thigh dominate the support phase. Your legs would collapse if the front muscles weren't dominating. The impossible attempt to push forward is the main reason for hamstring injuries.

THEIR ADVICE: Keep your shoulders from rotating.

MY RESPONSE: On the cover of the book in which this advice was written, there is a picture of the world's top marathoners. All of them have their shoulders rotated far around. A sprinter rotates the shoulders as hard as possible, but in very short turns. It is difficult and uncomfortable to rotate hard and short, but you can run faster that way. A distance runner doesn't require an exceptionally short shoulder rotation, but a sprinter does.

THEIR ADVICE: Develop a powerful forward thigh drive to increase your stride length, and then make a forceful leg pullback.

MY RESPONSE: Your foot needs to be driven with the same force as the thigh, down and forward. Delaying your foot return wastes time and energy. A forceful leg pullback—trying to push the body forward—will rip your hamstrings and won't even push back at the ground. You should never work at lengthening your stride. It slows you down.

The Big Guns of Running Advice Are Causing Mass Destruction

The advice of the standard running camps is patently absurd. My alternative biomechanics clearly demonstrates that the knee rotates in the opposite direction from what has been standard science until now. Nobody will argue that the knee rotates forward to toss the body up or that jumping action during running pushes your leg down and forward, not back and up as the standard science asserts. The muscles across the front of the knee (quadriceps) are used for that purpose. The leading scientific institutions teach the impossible science of pushing the foot against the ground, and making the stride long. Try it and you will see that the harder you push, and the longer you stride, the slower you will run. They can never acknowledge their mistakes because it will hasten their demise as leaders.

My Alternative Biomechanics Is Obvious.
It's Not Rocket Science.

The backward push that is taught never happens because the opposite action (forward push) is taking place and dominates. The muscles across the backside of your leg are used for a different purpose than pushing against the ground. These muscles are used to pull back your upper body as it lurches forward when your foot hits the ground.

The slanted leg, which is pushed by gravity, falls forward while it is jumping. If your weight stayed centered over your foot, you would jump straight up. Gravity pushes your leg forward when your weight is at a forward position in the rotation of your leg. Your leg takes the same action as a vaulting pole, except for the jump. Your foot is placed ahead of your body at landing, and your body's weight starts the vault from behind your foot and rolls forward ahead of your foot until your foot leaves the ground.

Gravity is simple science. When your weight is ahead of your toes, obviously you will be falling forward. No muscles can stop it or force it by pushing. It would be insulting your intelligence to ask you to wait for this to be scientifically proven.

Clarification of the Alternative Science

The runner whose feet drop farther back and more often to the rear than any of the other runners in a race always wins the event. Gravity pushes you harder, to fall forward faster, when your weight is positioned more toward the front, closer to the landing foot. Consider the following examples.

On a space station, you can jump up and go up forever, but you can't fall forward to walk or run. Your muscles are not positioned on your body to push you for the walking and running process. On the moon you would be able to run faster than on earth—if your legs could push you for that purpose. Gravity doesn't hold you back when you run, it is the starting and continuous force that powers the action. Everything you do with your muscles is reactive to the speed at which gravity pushes you. Because it is known that you can run faster on the earth than on the moon, why haven't any of the scientists figured out that it *must* be gravity that pushes you forward? Lighter gravity allows you to do everything easily with your muscles. You can jump higher and lift objects with less effort, but you can't run fast. The reason you can't run fast is because muscles can't push you forward...only gravity can. Lighter gravity, combined with momentum, pulls your body from behind your stationary foot to ahead of it much more slowly.

Try pushing forward when you are running backward and feel your muscles pushing forward at the ground. Then try pushing backward while running forward, and you can see that you can't push. It's because your legs can only push forward in either direction when you are standing on the ground. The quadriceps work both ways. You do not stop yourself from running by pushing forward because you roll on your foot.

When you are running on a treadmill, scientists haven't been aware of what keeps you aligned with the stationary frame of the treadmill. You are running ahead of the belt at a steady pace because your feet are dropping at the same angle to your weight with every landing. Drop your feet more to the rear, and you will pick up speed and hit the front of the treadmill. Drop your feet more to the front, and you will lose speed and move to the rear. Your sense of balance will eventually adjust the position of your weight for gravity to push you at a steady pace. Knowing the Nirenstein "Guided Muscles" way to adjust your balance for increasing speed will make it easy to accomplish.

What It Takes to Become Proficient with the Alternative Technique

You will be disillusioned when you first try this technique. Dropping your feet far back to zoom ahead much faster than you ever have won't happen to the degree that you might expect. Your sense of balance won't let you fall, so it will tighten your muscles and limit your progress to only a slight increase at first. Eventually you can progress much farther than ever before. But that will only be possible if you learn about additional factors that will help it happen. The following instructions are what you need to know:

1) How muscles move the body, and how they do so without interference from redundant muscles on the opposing side of joints.

2) How to exchange your feet quickly with a body twist, providing the power for the swing speed you need for pace.

3) How to angle your upper body for speed while causing the least strain on your muscles.

4) How to push yourself hard while staying within safe and optimal boundaries.

5) How to handle feelings of numbness and tension that are tied to the running process.

6) How to automatically get the most oxygen through muscle control.

7) How to lift off, stride, and land in ways that make the motion soft, smooth, fast, relaxed, and rhythmic.

If you miss any one of the features in this book, it could derail you. Each instruction is very significant to include in your technique for efficiency.

Intelligently Guiding Muscles for Improved Power with Relaxation

It is natural to be tense and uncoordinated in your movements and still look like you are emulating the movements of a champion athlete. Just because you've practiced and made natural adjustments to move your body in the same way as an elite runner doesn't mean you are applying the power properly. Your natural movements might use your energy to apply isometric contraction of your muscles. One muscle is pressed against another and little or no movement takes place. The improvements you make to your natural movement might not seem comfortable at first, but through repetition they will become natural and more comfortable. So instead of trying to just do it naturally, you need to Just Undo It first. Get rid of bad physics and improve the good. Many people know how muscles contract to move the body, but they don't know how to apply pressure to one side of a joint while totally loosening the ones on the opposite side. It is now possible to do that with what I call the "Guided Muscles" technique. We will start with the way your muscles move your limbs in a simplified way.

We will start out with the quadriceps muscle that crosses the front of the knee. It is attached to the front of the thighbone, crosses the knee, and attaches to the shinbone. A muscle can only be made to contract (shorten) to rotate a joint. It cannot be made to lengthen itself. When this muscle on the front of the knee shortens, it draws the front surfaces of the upper and lower legs closer together, extending the leg from a bent position. To command this muscle to contract for running, you have to guide it to apply pressure to the hip and to the

20

ground. You can get the most power (and speed) when you push off of an immovable platform (the ground) at one end of the leg, while the opposite end (the hip) is free to move through the air.

For the most speed, there must be the greatest possible force continuously applied between the endpoints of your leg to create the greatest resistance to your movement. That may be hard to understand in light of what you have been told about staying relaxed. The fact is, to produce your greatest power, you need to contract the right muscles as hard as you can, while at the same time totally relaxing all of the redundant muscles. (The opposing muscles that should be relaxed make up most of the muscles in the body.)

You are ready to apply your greatest force to jump. Here's what you need to do: The action for jumping is all in the leg. You need to contract the quadriceps muscles as hard as you can to straighten the leg. To do it effectively, you need to apply the most pressure you can feel against the hip at one endpoint and the ground at the other end. When you feel that pressure correctly, it will feel as if you are being completely stopped in your effort to jump by an equally strong resisting force. This is because you are being equally resisted. As Newton's Third Law states, for every action, there is an equal and opposite reaction. To practice tossing the body up, do these two exercises. First, jump as high as you can while tightening all of your muscles. Second, jump as high as you can by tightening the muscles across the front of the knee (quadriceps) and feel the heavy pressure between the foot and the hip. At the same time, loosen the rest of your muscles. This will teach you how to relax your opposing muscles.

The opposite and equal action does not come from the weight of your body alone. The leg push is strong enough to move your body. The weight of your body combined with the speed of it being pushed up causes the strong equal and opposite action. The pressure to overcome the inertia of your body, to resist adding speed, must be continued at full pressure for the length of the jump. In this way, speed will keep increasing exponentially for the length of the swing. Equal pressure must be felt on the opposite end of the leg, against the ground. Since your leg cannot move the ground, all of the power goes into lifting your body. The same scenario applies to lifting your heel by using the calf muscles in the latter stage of the jump.

The force it takes to raise the body should not be applied maximally for distance running. The stride should not be forced to shorten as strongly as in a sprint. A comfortable medium length stride is easier and more appropriate for distance running. In a sprint, your foot has to leave the ground faster to keep the spread of the feet shorter. Landing on your toes for sprinting helps accomplish that.

Exchanging the Feet Fast Via a Body Twist

The slower you exchange your feet, the slower your forward movement. It is necessary to put power into swinging your foot forward. When you walk you have time to bring your foot forward to land before your foot in back leaves the ground. When your speed becomes too fast for your leg to come forward in time to have both of your feet on the ground, your sense of balance tightens your muscles. You cannot increase speed unless you give yourself more time to exchange your feet by jumping with both feet in the air. The reason you become airborne when you run is to give yourself more time to exchange your feet. Your feet are forced to spread farther apart as you run faster by the speed differential between your body moving forward and the ground moving behind you. The larger spread of your feet in a faster pace does not send your raised foot further forward; it just sends your foot that is traveling behind you further back and up. While the foot is swinging forward faster to return, it is traveling a longer distance. For this reason, the exchange cannot be faster than at a slower speed and shorter stride.

The body twist locks the hip so that the foot and the opposite shoulder pressing forward can't rotate it. The foot going forward presses the hip from the front, while the opposite shoulder going forward presses the hip from the rear. That makes the hip an immovable platform from which both sides can push off with progressive speed. Both foot and shoulder meet greater resistance when speed increases and it also applies more pressure to the hip from opposite sides. The upper arm, when swung forward, adds resistance against the hip to allow greater force to swing the foot forward. In a distance run, the forearm is kept horizontal for comfort, and it does not contribute to the foot exchange. The hand and forearm should bounce loosely and not swing up and down. Again, this is in longer distance runs. In sprints, the lower arm is brought down and swung hard to add resistance against the hip so that the foot can be swung forward faster. In distance running the twist is longer and easier than it is in sprinting. In sprinting, the twist is very short and powerful. Keeping the arms swinging straight ahead does not affect the body twist. Runners do just as well turning their arms as they do driving them straight ahead.

Exchanging the feet faster does not increase your speed. Instead, it allows you to shift your body farther ahead on your landing foot. Gravity pushes you faster when your weight remains more to the front of your range of motion in the vault. Your sense of balance will tighten you up if your landing foot will not return fast enough to keep you from falling.

How to Lift off the Ground Properly When Running and Land in Ways That Make the Motion Softer, Smoother, Faster, More Relaxed, and More Rhythmic

When running at a steady pace, if you want to increase your speed, you must alter your landing spot, which is what holds you at your pace. You have to actually drop your feet behind your weight and keep them dropping behind until you want to level off. The only way you can increase speed with each step is to keep landing your feet behind your weight. Gravity and momentum add speed with each step, and that keeps you from falling. To level off at the faster speed, drop your feet ahead of your body, but not as far ahead as when you were at a slower pace. The more you drop your feet to the rear, the faster you will be running. It is impossible to see your exact landing spot, but it isn't necessary; you can feel yourself dropping your feet more to the rear. To feel how fast you are running, notice how high your feet are being flipped to the rear by the speed. The faster the speed, the higher your feet will be flipped by the speed differential between your body moving forward and the ground being left behind.

Your knee should be slightly bent for landing to avoid crushing it and to set your leg in position for lifting your body. The lift should be just high enough to keep your body level with the ground as your leg is spinning forward. With very little up and down motion, running is faster and more fluid.

To make running even more fluid with less impact, extend your stride in the air and return your foot backward before your land. This can be clearly seen in the fuller over-stride of a cheetah running at seventy miles an hour. The front feet over-stride high in the air and then take a long and fast swing back before the cheetah lands under its shoulders. The best physics does not return your feet faster than the speed of the ground moving away from you. The best physics enables you to land with the same speed as the ground moving away, so that you are standing neutral—without pushing or pulling. The angle at which your feet land—foot-to-weight position—will give you the amount of push from gravity.

The part of the foot you land on adds to softness and speed. For distance running, the best part of the foot to land on is the flat of the foot. The two pads in front of the arch and the pad behind the arch will absorb the shock better than landing on your heel. Your toe will also stabilize your foot better than your heel. It will keep it from rolling from side to side. Your foot does not have to be constantly rolling forward and side-to-side. The rolling should be done by your ankle until it is time to get up on your toe.

Many runners feel the illusion of landing on their heels, when they are actually landing flat. Especially if you are not jumping high, because you would trip if the toe were hanging low as your foot comes forward. When your toe is raised to avoid tripping, the touchdown starts lightly with the front part of the heel. The toe drops before the weight is fully on the foot, so the landing is actually flat. A sprinter gets more speed by landing on the toes. Your foot needs to lift off faster when your body is pulling away faster. Starting on your toe is faster than starting flat. Landing on your toes would be more efficient for the distance runner too, but the stress on the calf muscles would be too great. The foot is at a right angle to the leg, so the leverage against the calf muscles is great.

A major cause of hamstring injury is the strong effort runners use to push back at the ground. Nobody ever succeeds in actually pushing back. The jump takes place for the whole time your foot is on the ground. Jumping rotates your knee joint forward. This pushes your foot down and forward, so the effort to push your foot back is wasted energy. You should land as if you are going to be standing still. Let gravity do all the work of sending you spinning forward.

Keeping your feet pointing straight ahead will prevent injuries to the knees and other joints and muscles. If your hips are allowed to turn, your feet will turn with them. Make sure your hips stay square. If your leg is misaligned, you may have to get it corrected.

Locking your knee while the foot is high in the air and then dropping your body and foot hard shocks your knee joint severely. Your foot should be lowered to touch the ground softly while your body is in suspended animation. After contact is made with the ground, let your body press down. That way the impact will be eliminated.

Properly fitting orthotics are a must for protecting the bottom of your feet, correcting abnormalities, and softening the landings.

Correct posture will help reduce strain and open circulation and respiration.

How to Angle Your Upper Body for Speed and the Least Strain on Your Body

The best posture for running is the same posture for standing still. Essentially, the object is to let your body frame do as much of the work as it can to support your body and lighten the load on your muscles. Surprisingly, holding your upper body erect or tilting it at a forward slant does not shift the weight of your body from being centered over your feet. You can shift a vertical upper body as well as a forward-slanted upper body to the front of the feet and fall forward, or you can shift them behind your feet and fall backward.

Shifting your weight is not done by pushing with your muscles. When you are standing still, your weight is centered between your heels and toes. Lift your toes and your weight is now ahead of your heels. Gravity is exerting its downward force against a forward-slanted leg. The exerted force of gravity, acting against the reactive force from the slanted leg, spins your body forward. When you jump while falling forward, it keeps your body level with the ground.

For a distance run it is best to keep the upper body posture as vertical as when the body is standing still. Your torso can be shifted by putting a slight arch in your lower back to get better support from the spine. The spine is not located in the center of your torso, so a lot of weight remains in front of the spine. If you don't shift your torso back, the weight will curve your spine forward, and your shoulders will be rounded. When your torso is shifted slightly back, it remains balanced with the spine, and this balance reduces the stress on your muscles. Your shoulders will naturally stay back and not crunch your chest. It is

28

easier to breathe, and you get better circulation this way. Your shoulders should bottom out, rather than being pulled up in an impossible attempt to make your body lighter.

You will be able to improve your speed right away by knowing that your feet must be dropped further behind you. The initial increase will be marginal, though, until you develop a feel for shifting your body farther forward. Shifting your body forward has the same effect as dropping your feet more to the rear. You don't have any way to shift your body. Gravity does it when you position your feet off center. Other factors need to be developed as well: muscle strength, open circulation channels, a stronger diaphragm, and better coordination.

A sprinter should take the first couple of steps differently than a distance runner. You can double the speed of your first couple steps by jumping forward when your body is very low and your legs are very bent. In that position, straightening your legs with the quadriceps muscles will push you straight ahead. After a couple of steps, your running speed becomes faster than you can jump, so you have to rise up and continue to drop your feet to the rear. These first couple steps are important to getting a head start. The speed builds exponentially with each step, so the faster the start, the more help it will give you with your speed down the line.

Tilting Your Upper Body Is Not a Weight-Shift for Controlling Pace at All. You Can Run Just as Fast with an Erect Body as You Can with a Tilted Body

Where you drop your feet in relation to the center of your body determines your pace. You can tilt the body forward to a horizontal position and run backward if you drop your feet far in front of the center of your body. Keeping your body in a constant erect position is best for controlling pace, and for less stress on the back muscles as well.

Your feet automatically continue to drop at the same spread ahead of your body's center when you tilt the upper body forward, so your pace remains the same as when you held your body erect.

An erect upper body is supported more by your body frame and less by your muscles. The body rests comfortably on your leg. The rotations of your legs are free to move easily too.

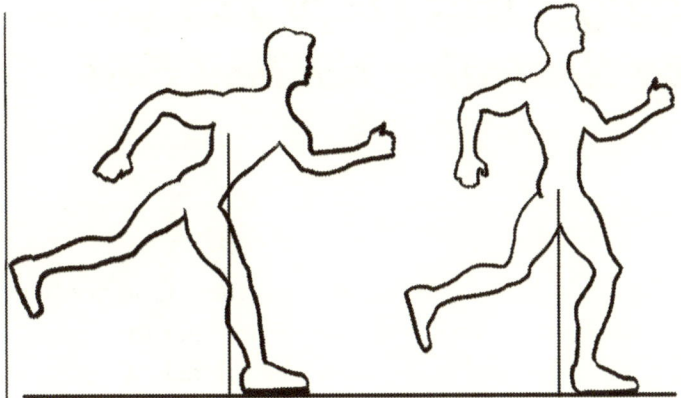

The Body Twist Helps You Go Fast by Returning the Feet Fast

When your body quickly flies forward, the returning foot needs to move out front in time to catch your body. Swinging your foot quickly forward is done by locking your hip so it can't be rotated. When your foot is pushed forward off of an immovable hip, more power can be used to swing your foot. Your right shoulder and left foot push off your hip from opposite sides and lock the hip and keep it from rotating. Your arms are part of the body twist and add additional force against your hip. It doesn't matter if your arms turn in across your chest or move straight forward; the same force can be used either way. Another reason why you shouldn't rotate your hip is because doing so turns your foot sideways and can injure your muscles. Jump in place and do the twist while you are in the air. Feel how you can drive your foot forward with power from the twist action.

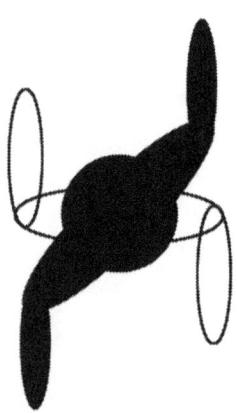

Eight Ways to Make Running Softer, Smoother, Faster, More Relaxed, and More Rhythmic

1. Don't push against the ground.
You can push back against your leg, but your foot can't press back against the ground. Your leg is pushing down and forward to toss your body up. When you make an attempt to push back against the ground, you can injure yourself severely.

2. Over-stride, then drop the foot down and back.
If you land on ground that is moving backward, the impact to your joints will be severe. To soften the landing, overstride and, while still in the air, drop your foot back to match the speed at which the ground is moving behind you.

3. Reach down and back.
While both feet are in the air and your body is in suspended animation, reach down and back with your front foot to touch the ground softly. When you touch the ground before your body drops, you will not smack into the ground.

4. Land flat.
Your toe should be raised when your leg is brought forward to avoid tripping. When you drop your foot, touch down softly with the flat of your heel, then let your toe drop down to catch the full weight of your body. This causes the impact to be absorbed across the front and back pads of your feet.

5. Land with your knee bent.
Landing with a straight leg crushes your knee. A bent knee can bend with the force.

6. Keep your body erect.

You can run just as fast with an erect body as you can with a tilted one by landing closer to your body's center of gravity. Your weight cannot be shifted any other way than by the angle of your leg when it lands. Gravity and momentum do all of the shifting by pulling your body down and forward. An upright body is supported by your body frame, so it's easier on the muscles.

7. Don't jump high.

The object of the jump is to counter your falling body with a toss-up that keeps you level with the ground. Any extra height wastes time and energy, and it slows the run.

8. Keep your feet pointed straight ahead.

When your foot is turned sideways at landing, your joints don't track properly. *Drop your foot behind you at the same speed that the ground is being left behind you, then let the ground drag your foot back and flip it up. This eliminates the impact and resistance.*

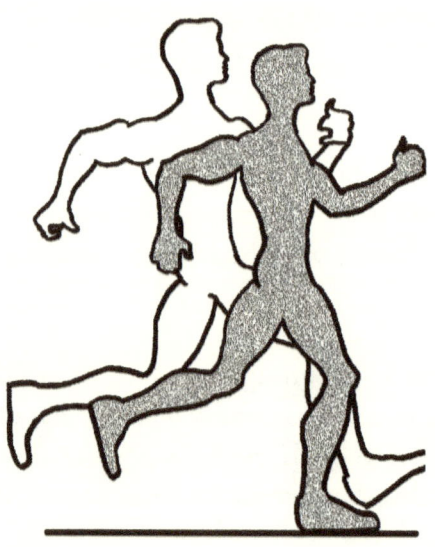

The Vaulting Process of the Legs Carrying the Body Forward Was Never Understood

Your feet do not have wheels that can move forward with your body. Your foot stands motionless on the ground while the top of your leg never stops going forward. The top of your leg begins the support phase from behind your foot and continues to move ahead of your foot before taking to the air. The shifting or vaulting of your body weight is never caused by a mechanical force from your body. *Gravity* exerts the pulling force, according to the landing angle of your leg. After the landing, the forces you apply are reactive to the speed at which gravity propels you. You have to time how long you stay on the ground, how fast you bring your leg forward, and how fast you push your body up. It isn't complicated to do this. You should take a medium stride length, one that feels comfortable for holding the pace.

Your body cannot stay still when your weight is ahead of the supporting foot, even though you are just standing without pushing.

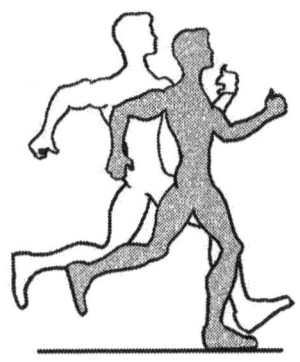

The runner changes positions during the support phase.

Position A: *He is standing without pushing back. Momentum is keeping him moving forward against the resistance from gravity. This is the last stage of the slowdown phase, which starts when his foot leaves the ground.*

Position B: *With the rest of his body now ahead of his foot, gravity and momentum are pulling him forward via his slanted leg.*

Position C: *The jump only raises him straight up. His body is pulled forward by gravity. The lift should be low, to reduce up and down movement.*

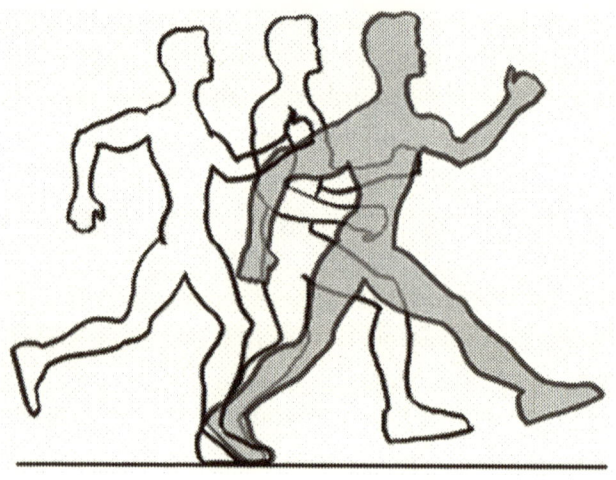

Changing Paces Easily and Knowing Your Speed

The only way you can change your pace is by altering the reach at which your foot steps down. Reaching far ahead slows the momentum so your body is slow when it moves directly over your foot. Once your body moves from behind your foot to over your foot, you've completed the slowdown phase. The slow momentum is combined with gravity to make you fall more slowly than if you had faster momentum. With a shorter reach, momentum is not slowed as much, so gravity and momentum produce more speed in the acceleration phase ahead of the vertical position.

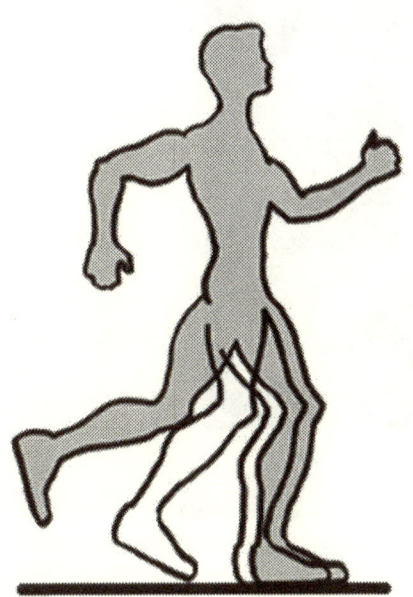

How Muscles Move Limbs

A skeletal muscle crosses a joint and attaches to two parts of the body on one side. It has a counterpart muscle on the opposite side that does the same thing. They work as a pair; one side shortens while the other side relaxes to lengthen. The purpose of your muscles is to create movement by shortening itself, which brings the body parts on its side closer together. When your muscles on the front of the leg are shortened, the lower leg moves forward. When your muscles on the back of the leg are shortened, the lower leg moves backward. If you shorten both sides simultaneously, no movement takes place. The leg is locked when the pressure to shorten is equal on both sides.

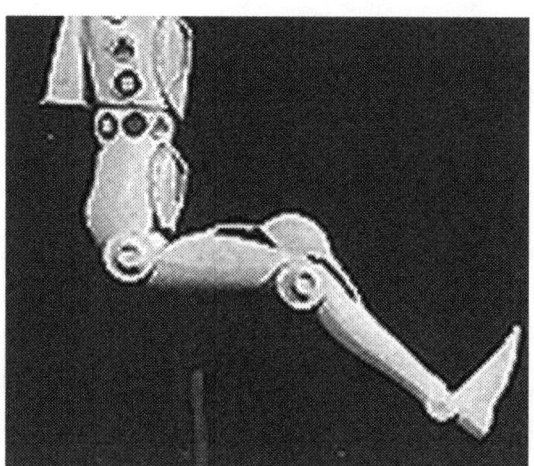

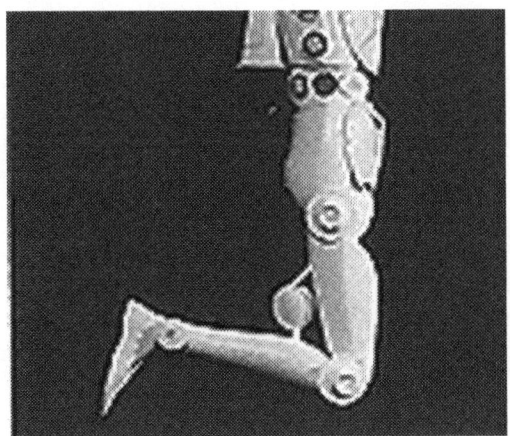

Here you see muscles on opposite sides working in pairs. The front thigh muscle (quadriceps) is shortening itself to move the lower leg's front side closer to the upper leg's front side.

Meanwhile, the muscle with which it is paired—located on the opposite side of the leg (hamstrings)—is relaxing for free movement. You should never shorten both sides at the same time.

When a muscle contracts itself (shortens), it is called *concentric contraction*. When a weight lengthens the muscle, but the process is slowed by the lightness of contraction, it is called *eccentric contraction*. Picture your lower leg moving down, but it is slowed in its descent by the quadriceps shortening themselves with lighter power than the weight of your leg. The net result is the lengthening of a muscle that is trying to shorten. The hamstrings remain relaxed.

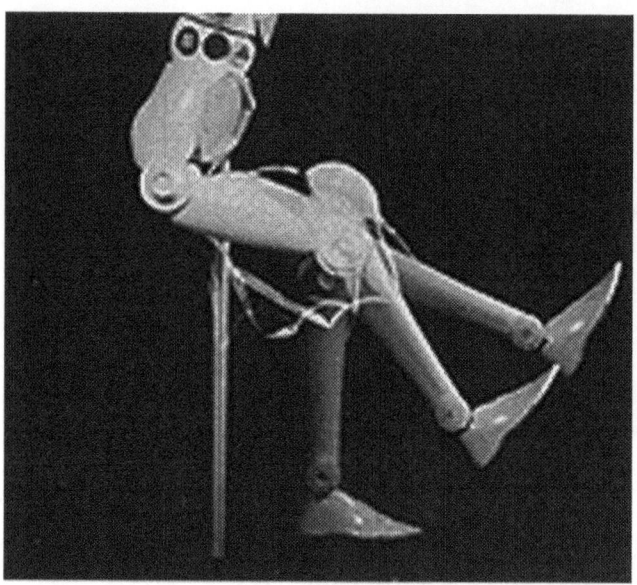

Body parts can move without muscles doing the work. Shown below: The lower leg was pushed down by gravity. It lengthened the front thigh muscle, which offered no resistance to its speedy descent. Its pair on the other side did not shorten itself by bulging. Gravity pushed the back of the lower leg closer to the back thigh.

It is very important to know how muscles move limbs, so that you can't be swayed by somebody's faulty logic. They've thrown terms at me, like *eccentric contractions*. They used it without explanation of how it applied. They didn't realize it didn't apply in the incident they were talking about.

Of course you couldn't move efficiently without this basic information. Every detail given in this book must be incorporated, or its efficiency will be lost.

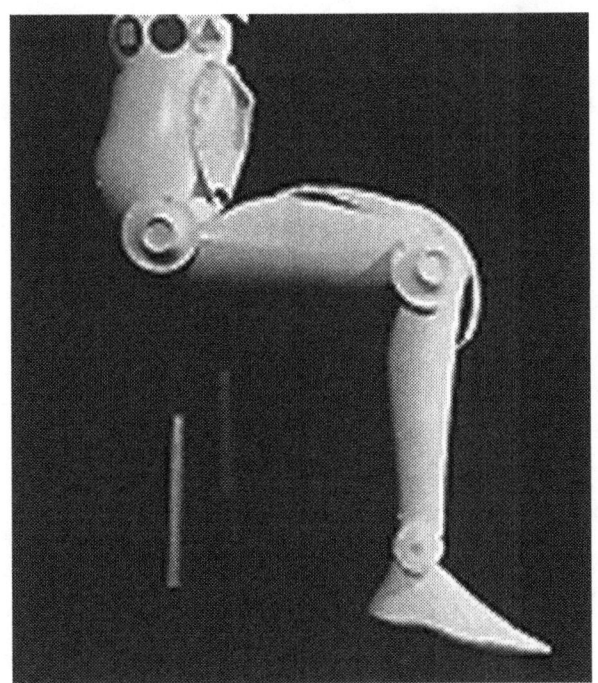

How Muscles Are Directed to Produce the Most Swing Speed

It seems odd, but the more resistance from inertia that you feel against the forward-moving muscle, the more speed will develop. In other words, the closer your muscle comes to the end of its power for moving the body part, the more it will release the free end of the leg from the resistance of inertia. Feeling the pressure build at the endpoints is your guide for contracting the muscle. The more pressure you feel the more speed will develop. You can get a better feel for directing the pressure if you pretend that you are pushing the atmosphere and it is resisting.

The longer the full pressure can be maintained, the more speed will develop. You have to be able to isolate one muscle from its pair on the opposite side of the joint. You can learn to do that by alternately using the opposing muscle to resist, then releasing it as much as possible for free movement. You will feel the extra speed develop.

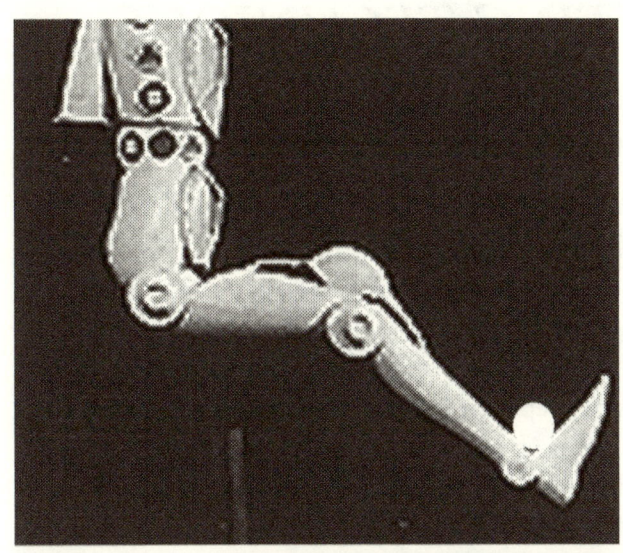

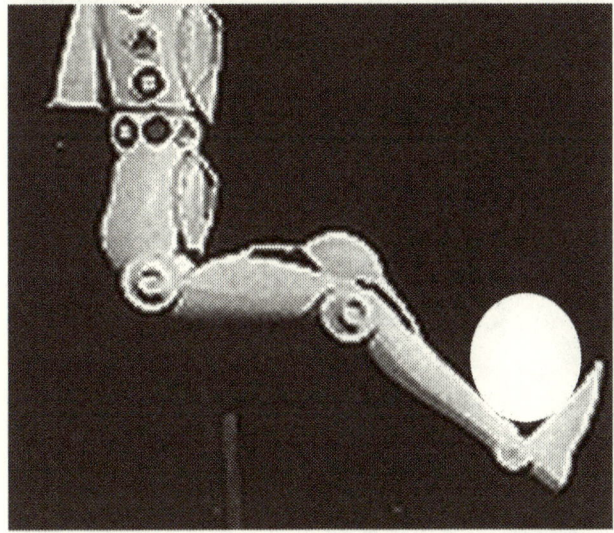

SPRINTING TECHNIQUE

A sprinter starts running with a technique that gives him a maximum push from gravity for the first two steps. It is similar to the way an animal starts to sprint. Gravity is pulling the hardest to make him fall forward when his weight is as far ahead of his feet as it can be. The legs lift the body when he falls to keep him level with the ground. This method is only good for two steps, because the weight cannot stay that far ahead of the feet for very long. The third and subsequent steps have to land closer to the body's center of gravity, but still behind it. Animals start sprinting by jumping with their front feet the same way a sprinter pushes up with his hands.

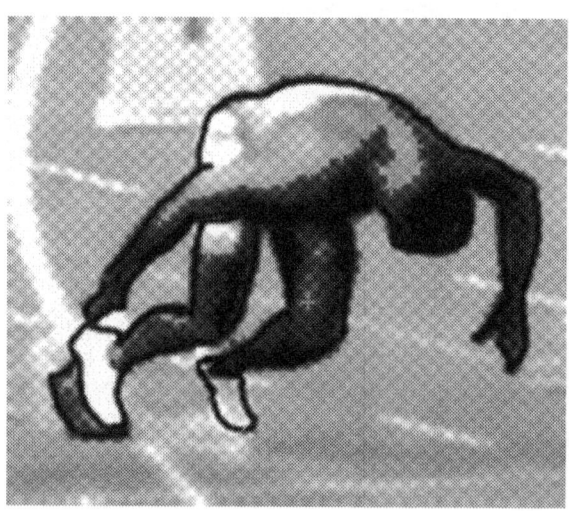

The back foot pushes off the block, sending the weight far ahead of the forward foot. The forward foot pushes off the forward block for the hardest pull from gravity. Since each step builds speed exponentially (for example, the second step is twice as fast as the first, etc.), any extra speed at the start gives the sprinter a decided advantage. The raised foot has to be brought forward as fast as possible in a sprint, in order for the weight to be caught for balance with the speed. The hard body twist against a non-rotating hip makes it happen. The stride in sprinting has to be kept as short as possible from start to finish of the sprint. That may come as a surprise, because the spread of the feet increases with speed. It can be easily explained. As the speed increases, the foot is dragged back faster by the ground. No matter how hard you work to keep the spread of the feet short, the speed will overcome your power and spread your feet farther apart. The shorter you keep the spread of your feet, the more your weight can be kept to the front for a harder push by gravity. The more resistance you feel to keep you from twisting, the faster you can exchange your feet. That is why a sprinter puts all of his effort into keeping the twist short and hard. He also lowers his forearm to add resistance to the twist. That way he can push the foot forward faster. Speed builds faster with more resistance to move, because speed buildup is added to the force of getting a heavy body moving.

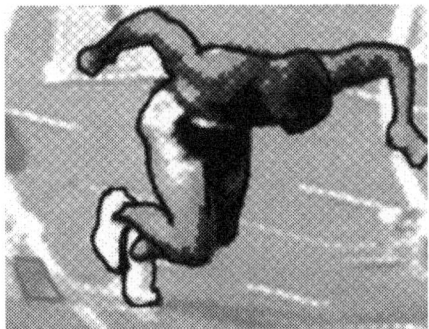

The third step shows the foot landing closer to the body's center of gravity. The shallower angle is an adjustment made to keep the body from falling to the ground. The feet can no longer be exchanged as fast as they were in the first two steps out of the blocks. The body must make an adjustment in balance, so it rises to reduce the strain on the back muscles. A tilted upper body does not put the weight any farther ahead of the foot than an upright upper body. You can run just as fast either way. The erect upper body puts less stress on the muscles to help you run more easily. It is impossible to see the exact spot at which the foot is fully pressed into the ground to start it vaulting forward at the hip. It isn't necessary to see the spot, because when you signal your feet to drop more to the rear, you can feel it happening. If you want to increase speed, just drop your feet more to the rear and it must happen. Gravity is going to push you harder when you start the fall from a more forward position.

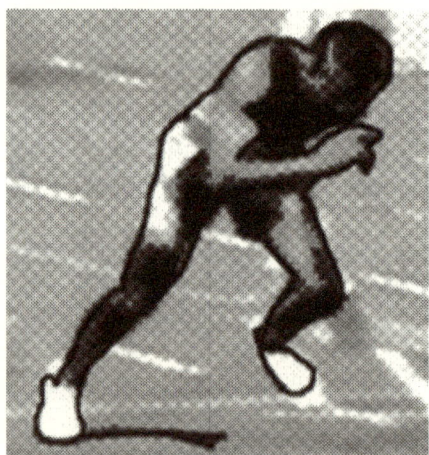

The sprinter takes many more steps with his feet dropping to the rear of his weight than a slower runner. The forward shift of his weight, combined with the extra steps at his angle, builds more speed. Here you see an over-stride that takes his foot ahead of the landing angle while in the air. His foot will drop back while his body flies forward and lands behind the weight. The over-stride and drop back is a very important technique to avoid impacting the ground hard against the speed. The drop back of the foot is not meant to be fast to push back against the ground. You should match the speed of the ground moving backward and stand neutral. Feel the ground pulling your foot back after you land and stand relaxed.

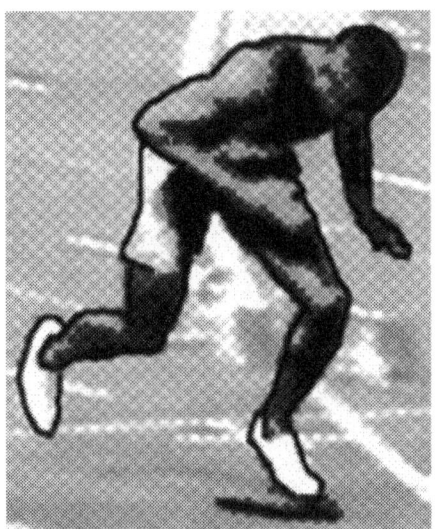

This picture shows the landing angle of the foot maintaining the position of landing behind the weight. The raised foot is flipped higher by the ground moving away faster. The same landing angle is maintained during the whole speed increase phase. When the maximum speed of the sprinter is reached, the landing position is changed to provide a level pace. The foot lands slightly ahead of the weight to produce a slight slowdown. Momentum carries the body past the foot, then momentum and gravity increase the speed just enough to match the slowdown from the landing. Less air time and shorter reach of your foot ahead of your weight give you the most speed.

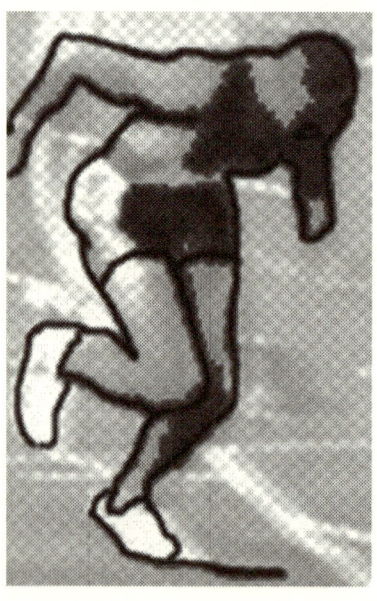

The grounded foot is dragged back with great force when the sprint is at full speed. The body falls far ahead of the foot, where it gets a hard push from gravity. The foot leaving the ground is held loose before the reverse direction can be fully implemented. As a result, the lower leg bends the knee and keeps the foot flying high. This wide spread of the feet is an unavoidable inefficiency in biomechanics. The feet should not be spread apart deliberately.

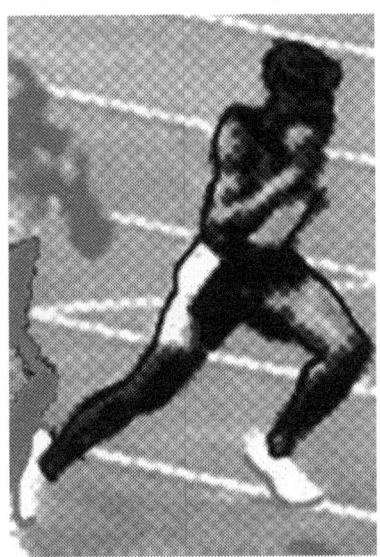

The spread of the feet is at its maximum, and the raised foot needs to be returned with the maximum speed possible. The longer distance the foot travels up, and the longer distance it has to return to land, makes for a slower exchange of the feet than is executed during a slower run. The swing of the leg is speedier in a sprint than in a slow run. The landing will take place with the foot positioned slightly ahead of the weight. To get the most speed, try to hold back the spread of your feet with your body twist, but shift your weight as far ahead as you can to gain the speed that will overcome your effort and make your foot go way up. With all of your effort being used to condense the spread of your feet, feeling the feet spread farther apart tells you how fast you are running.

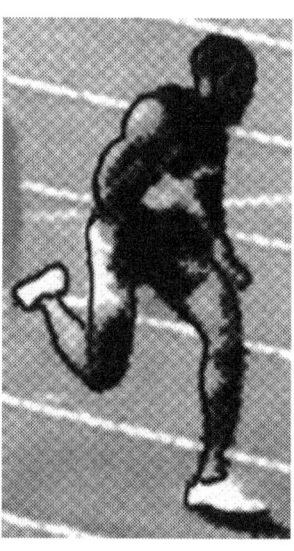

Combining All of the Techniques to Make You a Technologically Perfect Runner

You can begin learning scientific technique at any level of fitness, whether you run at a pace just slightly faster than a walk or at a championship speed. The first few techniques listed below will make running softer, smoother, and faster. You should start with two or three techniques and practice them for a week or two before adding one or two new techniques. Since neglecting any one of the many techniques can derail you, you won't be a completely efficient and safe runner until you incorporate them all into your running program.

1. No Push: Start running or walking at your normal, comfortable pace, using your natural technique. You don't have to understand what you have been doing, just do it. Now start the first technique: While you are moving along, stop all effort to push back at the ground to propel yourself forward. Notice that when you stop pushing, you do not lose any speed, and it becomes easier to move. Just standing and being pushed by gravity is what you have been doing all along, but now you are doing it with less tension. The part of your old technique that was pushing back did nothing to move you. It just tied you up, and was a prescription for injury.

2. Bent Knee: Add a second method while continuing with the first. Make sure your knee is slightly bent when you land. It will absorb the impact of the landing and avoid the crushing of the knee. A bent knee makes lifting easier.

3. Toss-Up: The third and last method of your initial training phase of the Guided Muscles technique is how to do the toss-up. Gravity only pushes straight down. Your leg won't let your body go straight down, so gravity spins your body downward and forward, spinning it around your foot as the axis. Straightening your leg to toss yourself up while falling keeps you falling straight ahead level with the ground, so you can continue running. Feel the pressure at the hip and foot when you shorten your muscles across the front of the knee for the toss-up. At the same time, loosen the muscles across the back of the knee that have been holding you back, to let the lift be easy. Do jumps in place while alternating between tightening all of your muscles and loosening all of the muscles except the quadriceps that rotate the knee forward. It will condition you for being relaxed. Don't jump high to stride long—short is better. Lift just enough to keep yourself level with the ground as your raised foot comes in for a landing with a slightly bent knee. Raise your toe to keep the forward-swinging foot from tripping.

4. Foot Plant: Raise your toe as you bring your raised foot forward to keep from tripping. Lightly touch the ground with a nearly flat heel. Let your toe fall freely just as your heel is starting to press. Allow the impact of the landing to be absorbed by the three pads of the foot. One pad is under the heel, and two are in front of the arch. This flat landing is what is best for all speeds except sprinting. In sprinting you must land on the two forward pads of the foot to get off the ground faster.

5. Back Drop of Foot: A slight over-stride with your forward-moving foot, followed by a back swing of the same foot as the foot lowers to the ground will lessen the impact and smooth your running. When starting a sprint, the speed is slow for the first few steps, so the spread of the feet is short. The flip back of your foot by the ground is but a matter of inches as your body moves ahead slowly. The spread of the feet continues to lengthen as the speed increases to full sprint, when your foot reaches your butt. The flip back becomes faster and faster as the speed increases, without any physical effort from the runner to bring the foot to the rear. The effort to reverse the direction of your feet cannot be implemented fast enough to keep your feet from spreading apart to a wide distance in a sprint. Both feet are forced to over-stride in opposite directions before being returned.

6. Reach Down, Touch Softly: While the forward foot is reaching back it should also be lowered to the ground. Make a soft touch to the ground with the foot before the weight of the body presses it fully.

7. Exchanging the Feet: Reversing the direction of the feet takes place when both of your feet are in the air. It requires a major effort from every joint in your body. The arms, shoulders, hip, and knee joints are rotated with equal force. The use of all your muscles is what makes running such a great exercise for health and fitness. Before you run, stand with your left foot forward and your right shoulder forward. Your body is standing in a twist position. Bend down and then jump up. While in the air, twist your body in the opposite direction so that your right foot is forward and your left shoulder is forward. Your hips are the center of the twist and do not rotate. The push to twist your upper body pushes off the back of your hip. The push to twist your foot forward pushes the front of your hip. Your hips are locked in place from pressure on both front and back and act as a solid platform from which to push off. Now run with the same kind of body twist you did in place.

8. Pointing the Feet: Point your feet straight ahead. Make sure your hip doesn't turn, because if it does, your foot will turn with it. If your legs are misaligned so that you can't land with your foot pointing straight ahead, see a doctor to correct it before you run.

9. Posture: The posture in running applies only to your upper body angle related to the vertical line of gravity, because your legs never stay at one angle under your body. The slant of your leg, not of your upper body, determines your speed. You can run at the same speed with your body erect as you can with your body tilted. In that case, the best posture for the upper body is the one that puts the least strain on your muscles. That position is an erect body. For many people, their spines tend to curve forward too much while they are standing erect. This is because there is a lot of weight in front of the spine and much less in the back. Putting a slight arch in the small of your back will center your chest in line with gravity and bring your shoulders back to a comfortable position in which they don't compress your chest. Put a slight arch in your neck to center your head as well. Now run while keeping the posture in mind.

10. Foot Placement for Pace: Your leg is locked at the joints for supporting your body's weight. It holds your body up as if it were a solid pole with no hinges and little flex. The placement of your foot is similar to where you would plant the bottom of a vaulting pole for a horizontal vault. Plant your foot far ahead of your body and you are vaulted high and become slowed down by the long swing of your body from behind your foot to the vertical position. Once past the vertical lift, the fall is slower because it is not accompanied by fast momentum, which was lost in the rise. Plant your foot closer to the vertical position of the leg, and you have a short rise time, which doesn't slow the momentum as much. When your body reaches the vertical, it has faster momentum to add to speedup the fall forward. Start running and maintain a slow pace. Notice how little your foot is flipped to the rear after it leaves the ground. This short flip back tells you that your pace is slow because you are reaching out far with your landing. Pick up speed by dropping your feet to the rear of your weight. You will increase speed with each step until you find the level of speed you wish to maintain. To level off and hold the faster pace you have reached, drop your feet ahead of your body at a different reach than the slow, steady pace. The reach has to be shorter from your body's center at a faster pace. Notice the higher flip back of your foot at the faster pace. The height of the higher flip tells you that you are running faster. Repeat the slow run, pick up speed, and level off to condition your sense of balance for adding speed.

11. Improving Agility: Stride length and foot speed are the professional standards of technique. These are not the right formula to improve agility. The right way is to improve your reaction time to start both the body twist and the lifting of the body. The rapid body twist condenses the spread of your feet. The rapid lifting of your body keeps your body on a more even keel. Power must be applied early and hard to speed both your foot return and lift.

The spread of your stride is lengthened by the running speed and limits your pace. So while you are swinging your feet faster and harder, you are not actually exchanging your feet faster.

The spread of your feet widens to the rear of your body. Your foot is flipped back higher by the speed of the faster pace. No effort should be made to pull your foot back and up. A shorter spread of your feet allows you to add more speed than a longer one.

Practicing rapid-fire exchanges of your feet—with body twists and body lifting—while coaxing your sense of balance—to allow you to drop your feet more to the rear—is the balance formula for speed.

Air time is slowdown time, so you want to shorten your air time. You can't do that by increasing the spread of your feet.

12. Pain Reduction: Your reaction to pain can increase its intensity or reduce it. You can cut the messages of pain flowing to your brain by tensing your entire body, but that adds swelling and eventually causes more intense pain. The best and healthiest way to reduce pain is through muscle control. This is where the Guided Muscles technique shines. It teaches you to separate your movement muscles from the anti-movement muscles. Anti-movement muscles are the muscles that move you in the opposite direction when they become the movement muscles. In running, the two main movement groups of muscles are the muscles that lift the body and the muscles that twist the body for exchanging the feet. Start running and feel the pressure between your hip and the ground when you contract the muscles across the front of your knee. While running, feel the front muscles between your hip and lower leg swinging your foot forward. Feel the pressure on the front muscles of your body on the opposite side—between the shoulder, arm, and the hip—that swing the arm forward. When you feel the pressure in the right areas for movement, you can fully release the pressure in the anti-movement areas. Start running again and don't concern yourself when your muscles press the swelling in your legs. With the reduction in tension, the blood will flow more easily, and the sensations of blood flowing and the correct muscles tensing will be more tolerable.

Breathing Technique

Located at the bottom of your rib cage is an umbrella-shaped muscle (diaphragm) that covers your lower stomach. It is held up by your lower stomach and is attached to your ribs. When your diaphragm contracts, it pushes the content of your lower body down, compressing it and expanding it somewhat. The lowering of your diaphragm draws air into your lungs. When the contraction of the diaphragm is released, the compressed lower stomach pushes your diaphragm back up and expels the air from your lungs.

This happens automatically, without any voluntary effort to force these muscles. Stronger breathing action can be achieved by deliberately and forcefully contracting the diaphragm while countering it with a stronger contraction of the lower stomach muscles. It is not worthwhile to force the breathing process. The automatic systems can bring in more air by being more rhythmic and by coordinating the compression and decompression better.

A focused effort should be made to keep your lower stomach muscles loose. That allows the diaphragm to go farther down and draw a full amount of air into the lungs. When the lower stomach muscles are held tight, the chest expands but less air is drawn in.

You can feel numbness and aching in your legs, but your breathing may be relaxed when your upper body is relaxed and the circulation channels are open. When your leg muscles get stronger, you can work the diaphragm harder and build up more breathing capacity.

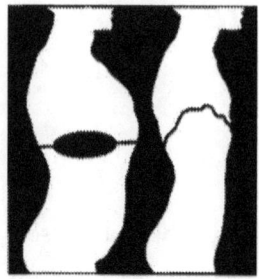

Technique for Building Muscle Strength with Weightlifting Designed to Increase Running Speed and Avoid Injuries

Overall strength in every muscle of your body will protect you from injury and help you increase your running speed. The popular method of lifting weights is not the best way for runners. The popular method of lifting weights is done by contracting the muscles on one side of a joint to move limbs and torso and at the same time resisting the movement with muscles on the opposite side. The resistance part of the lift trains the body to be tense for all movement.

When you apply my Guided Muscles technique to weightlifting, you train to add power with the strength. The power to create fast movement is developed by a method that adds more power to the pushing/pulling muscles and totally relaxes the opposing muscles. Muscles push the limbs or torso when they are Extended, and different muscles pull when they are bending them. In both instances, muscles flex (shorten) to bring the limb surfaces that are on the same side of the flexing muscle closer together. They push or pull the most when one endpoint is locked in place while the opposite end is free to move. The one endpoint can be locked by applying pressure against a rigid frame, the floor, or the back of an exercise bench. It can also be done by pulling the feet and torso together.

Weightlifting power is created by increasing the speed of the lift from start to finish. To do so, apply pressure against the two endpoints on the far sides of the two limbs that are connected by a joint. When doing a bench press, you should feel the pressure against the immovable bench at one end of the arm, and against the movable weight at the other end of the arm.

It is not the air that is causing the resistance to prevent the loose end of a limb from moving. You are pushing the weight of the body to move rapidly, while transitioning from a motionless stage to a speedy one. The inertia of your body acting against movement is what you feel holding you back. Keeping that in mind, the weight of your body combined with the inertia of ever-increasing speed is what is counteracting your push. The more resistance that you use to stop the movement, the more speed will increase. Heavy resistance felt throughout the entire length of a long swing will get you the greatest speed buildup.

Heavy weights won't allow you to move them beyond a small increase in speed. As long as you are flexing the movement muscle hard and totally relaxing its counterpart on the opposite side of the joint, you will get the training effect for speed.

To understand how heavy resistance gives you the most speed, try this (or just picture it in your mind): Lightly push a heavy punching bag, and you will find that there is little resistance against moving it. But with the slight power and resistance the bag wasn't building up speed as it moved for the length of the swing.

Now push the bag a little way forward and let it push your hand back. Stop the backward push of the bag with a forward push by your hand. An instant after starting the forward push, use all of the power you can muster to push the bag. This maintains the same maximum power until the end of contact with the bag. The bag keeps building speed throughout the swing until it reaches the maximum speed you can deliver to it.

The higher resistance you felt was from adding speed to pushing the bag. The more speed you add to push your body and an object, the heavier it becomes, which gives you more resistance. You can't ease off the movement muscles and achieve the same speed as you can with a harder push.

LEG EXTENSION

Position your knees in alignment with the machine's axis of rotation. Adjust the seat to support your back. Assume the starting position. Extend both legs simultaneously. Feel the pressure to move between the stabile endpoints at the bottoms of the thighs and the movable endpoints of the lower end of the shins. Do not lock out your knees. Press lightly to take up the slack in your relaxed muscles. Add power to move your ankle up. Maintain equal pressure for the rest of the swing. Return slowly to the starting position. Repeat in continuous motion without hesitation. Relax all muscles that are not straightening the leg by pressing the pad to move through space. Let the breathing be automatic without help from stomach muscles. (See "Breathing Technique.")

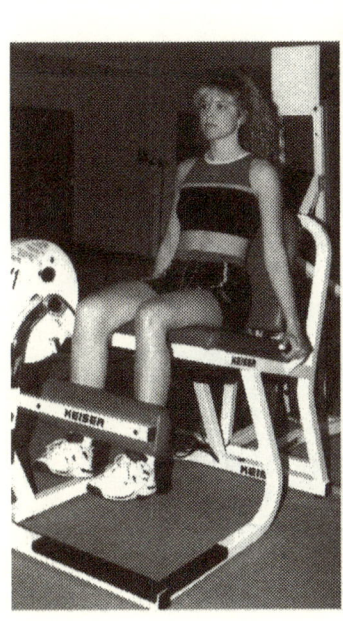
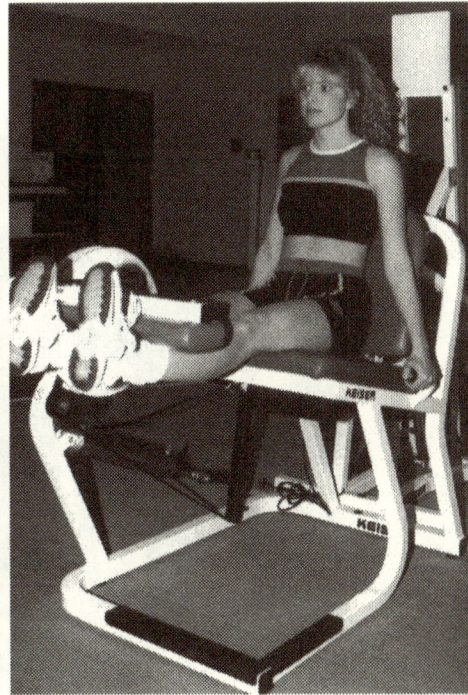

STANDING CALF

Stand on the front balls of your feet at the edge of the step. Place your hands in a comfortable position on the carriage. Keep your knees locked for the entire exercise. Keep your hips forward and your body in a straight line. Raise your heels as much as possible.

Feel the pressure move between the endpoints at toes and hip. Press lightly to take up slack in the relaxed muscles. Add power to move the hip up. Maintain equal pressure for the rest of the swing. Return slowly to the starting position. Repeat in continuous motion without hesitation.

The machine can be used similarly for squats with slight knee bends. This exercise gives extra strength for running. Keep your feet centered on the step between heels and toes. Relax all your muscles that are not straightening the leg by pressing the hip to move up. Keep your breathing automatic without help from your stomach muscles. (See "Breathing Technique.")

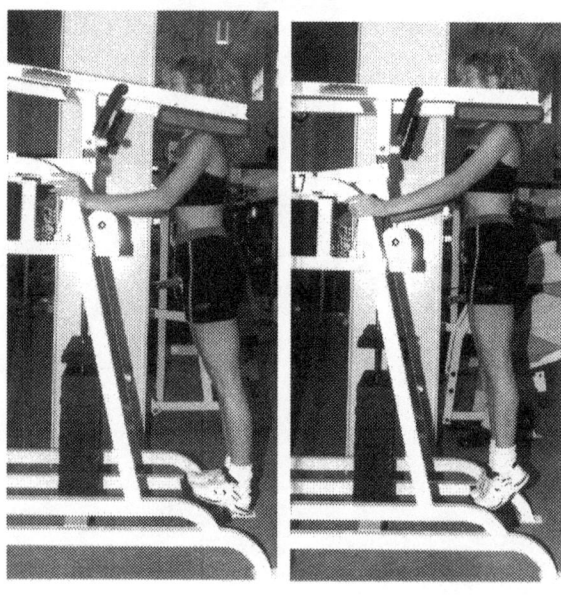

CHEST PRESS

Hold the handles with an open grip. Sit erect with your back fully resting against the pad and your spine slightly arched forward. Feel the pressure move between the stabile endpoints of your shoulders and the movable endpoints of your hands. Press lightly to take up slack in the relaxed muscles. Add power to move your hands forward at a slow speed. Maintain equal pressure for the rest of the swing. End the swing before you lock your elbow. Return slowly to the starting position. Repeat in continuous motion without hesitation. Relax all muscles (except those in your arms) and push forward through space. Keep your breathing automatic without help from your stomach muscles. (See "Breathing Technique.")

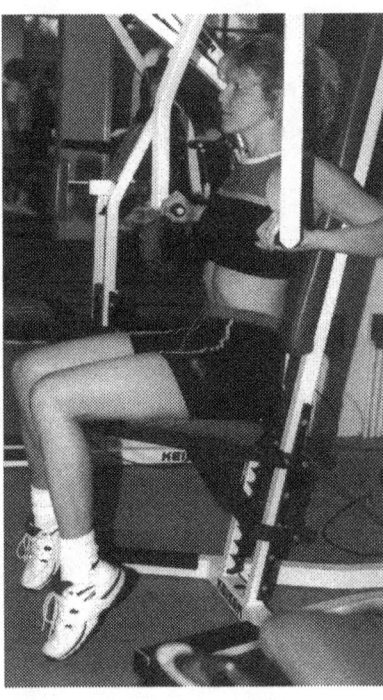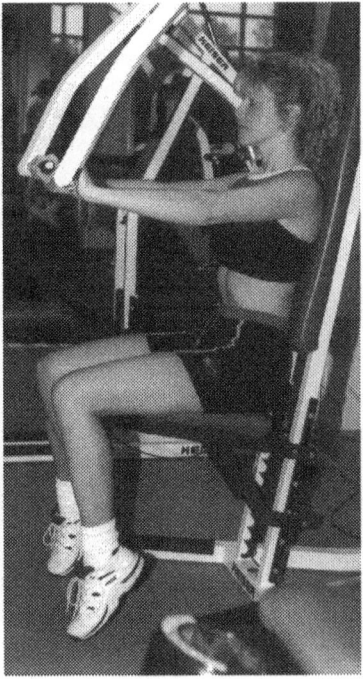

LOWER BACK

Press your feet flat against the platform. Feel the pressure move between the stabile endpoints of your feet and the seat and the movable endpoint of the upper back. Press lightly to take up the slack in the relaxed muscles. Add power to move your shoulder back at a slow speed. Maintain equal pressure for the rest of the swing. End the swing before your weight rests on the machine. Return slowly to the starting position. Repeat in continuous motion without hesitation. Relax all the muscles that are not pressing the shoulders back by pressing the pad to move it through space. Keep your breathing automatic without help from your stomach muscles. (See "Breathing Technique.")

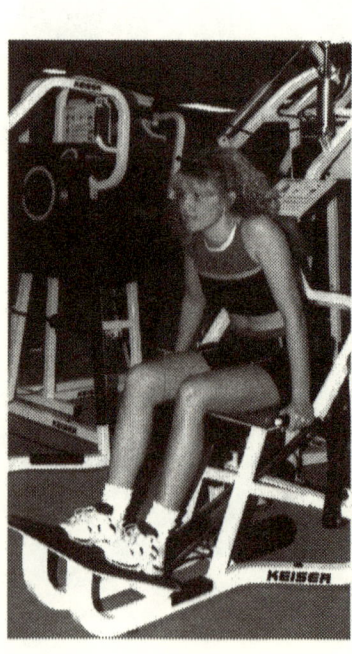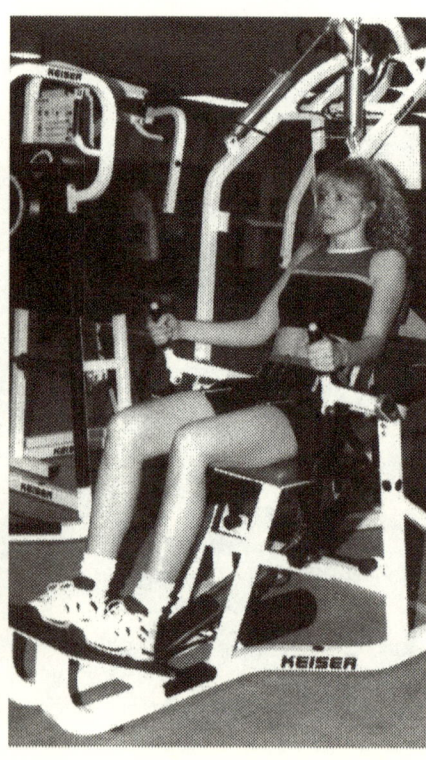

TRICEPS

Sit with your back fully resting against the back pad. Hold the handles with an open grip. Fasten the belt between your thighs and hips. Feel the pressure move between the stabile endpoints of your shoulders and the movable endpoints of your hands. Press the handles forward and down without locking your elbows. Return slowly to the starting position. Repeat in continuous motion without hesitation. Relax all muscles that are not pushing your hands forward and down by pressing the handles to move it through space. Keep your breathing automatic without help from your stomach muscles. (See "Breathing Technique.")

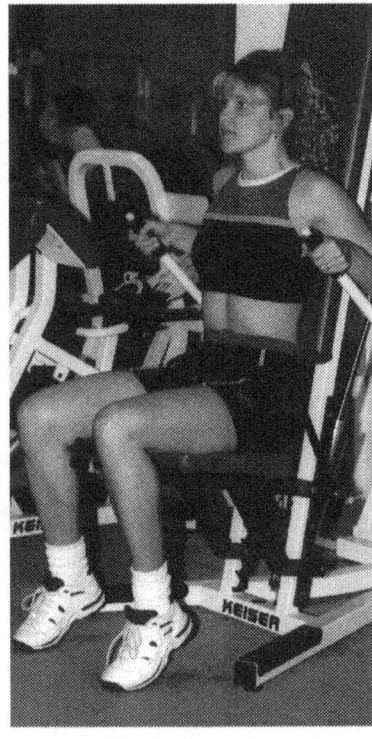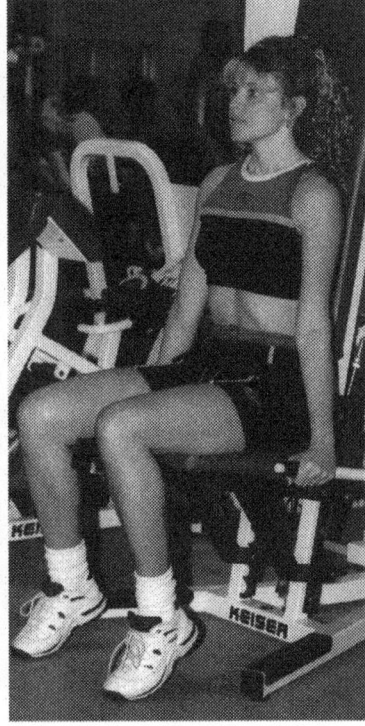

HIP ADDUCTION

Lean back, with your back fully resting on the back pad, place your feet on the foot pads, and your knees against the knee pads. Feel the pressure move between your stabile buttocks and your movable knees. Press your knees forward and inward to the limit. Return slowly to the starting position. Repeat in continuous motion without hesitation. Relax all your muscles that are not pushing your knees forward and inward by pressing the pad to move it through space. Keep your breathing automatic without help from your stomach muscles. (See "Breathing Technique.")

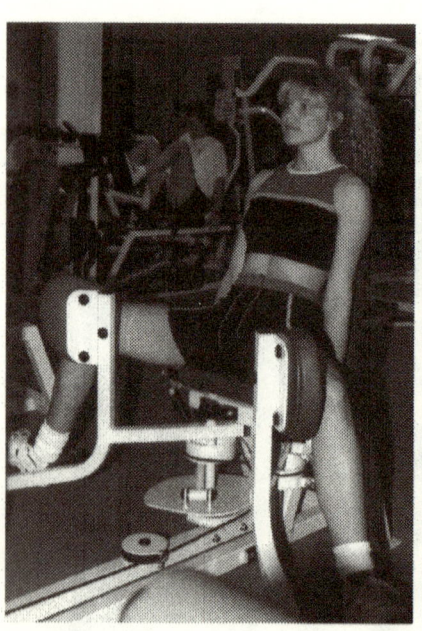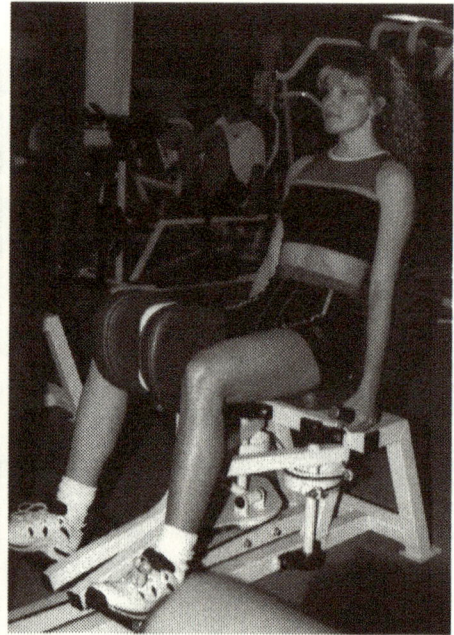

DIP CHIN ASSIST

Adding weight to the machine presses the knee pads up to help support your body weight. Hold on to the handles and place your knees on the pads. Slowly let your body drop. Do not lock your elbows. Press between the stabile endpoints of your hands and the movable endpoints of your shoulders. End the swing before your weight rests on the machine. Return slowly to the starting position. Repeat in continuous motion without hesitation. Relax all the muscles that are not pushing your shoulders up. Keep your breathing automatic without help from your stomach muscles. (See "Breathing Technique.")

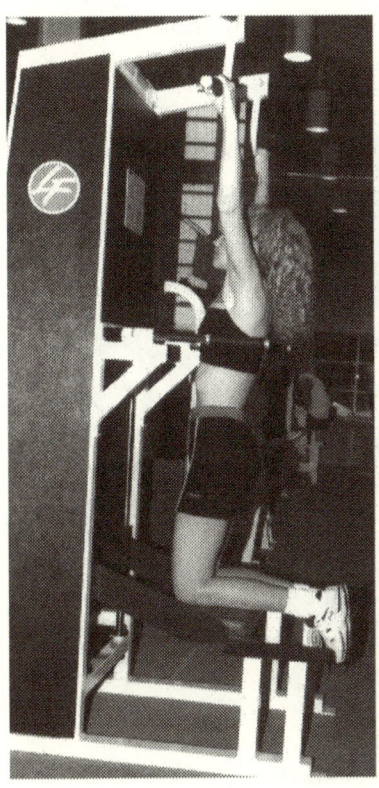
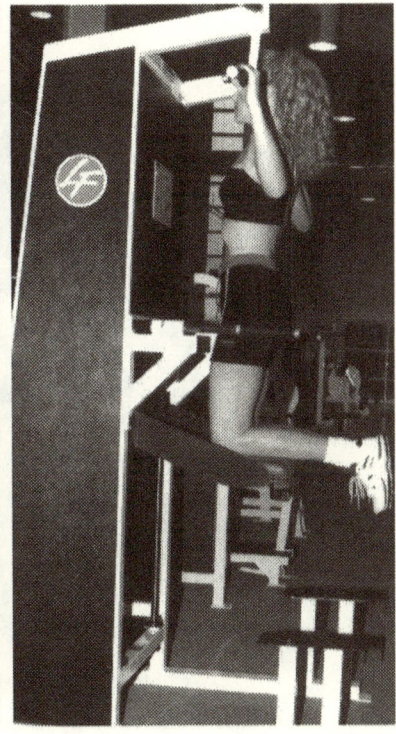

TRICEPS

Adjust the seat so that your elbows line up with the axis of the machine's rotation. Hold the handles with an open grip. Feel the pressure move between the stabile endpoints of your buttocks and arms (against side and underarm pads) and your movable hands. Start the swing with your hands slightly behind your elbows and end it with your hands halfway past your elbows. Press lightly to take up slack in your relaxed muscles. Add power to move at a slow speed. Maintain equal pressure for the rest of the swing. Return slowly to the starting position. Repeat in continuous motion without hesitation. Relax all your muscles that are not pushing your hands forward and down by pressing the handles to move them through space. Keep your breathing automatic without help from your stomach muscles. (See "Breathing Technique.")

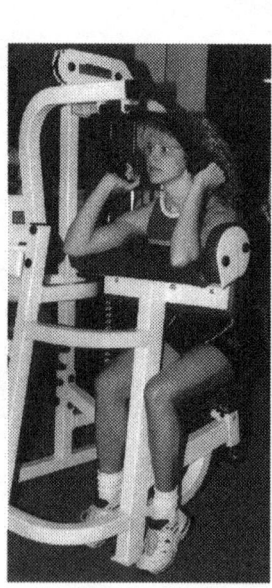
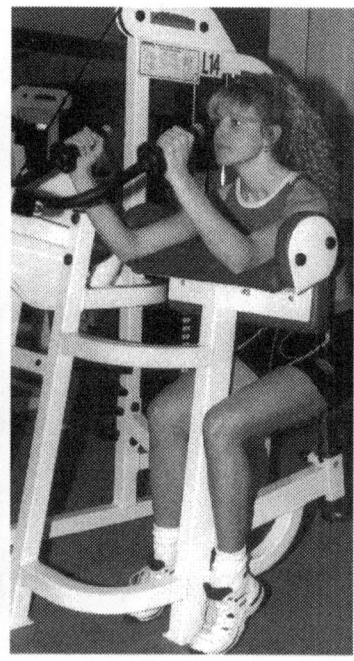

LAT PULL DOWN

Hold the handles at either end of the bar, lean forward, and bring the bar down to the back of your neck or upper shoulders. Return to the starting position. Do not lock your arms. Feel the pressure move between the endpoints of your stabile shoulders, thighs, and feet at one end and your movable hands at the other end. Another exercise consists of bringing the bar down to the front of your shoulders. Press lightly to take up slack in your relaxed muscles. Add power to move at a slow speed. Maintain equal pressure for the rest of swing. Return slowly to the starting position. Repeat in continuous motion without hesitation. Relax all your muscles that are not pulling your elbows down by pressing your hands to move the bar through space. Keep your breathing automatic without help from your stomach muscles. (See "Breathing Technique.")

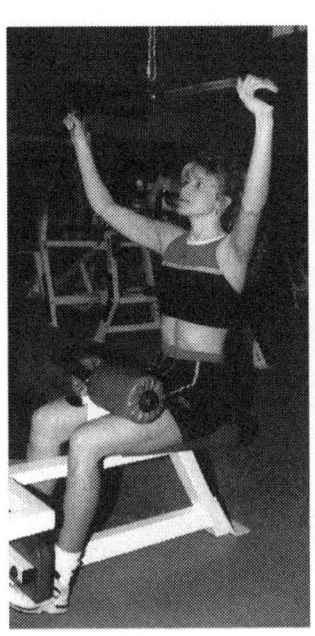
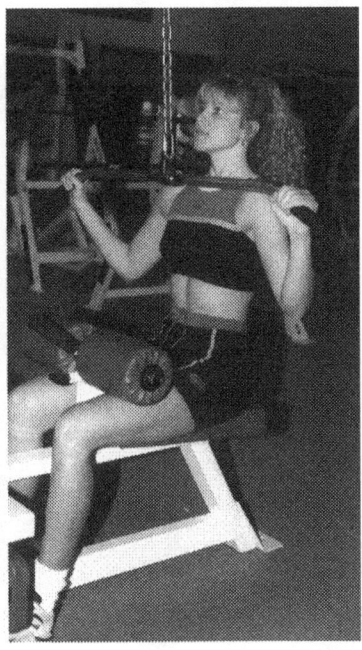

ABDOMINAL

Adjust the seat height to line up between the bottom of your chest and the top of your hip with the marker on the machine. Hold the handles with an open grip. Push the front balls of your feet against the frame. Bend halfway down. Feel the pressure move between the stabile endpoints at your feet and buttocks and the movable endpoints of your shoulders. Return slowly to the starting position. Feel the pressure move between the endpoints of your ankles and shoulders. Press lightly to take up slack in your relaxed muscles. Add power to move at a slow speed. Maintain equal pressure for the rest of the swing. Return slowly to the starting position. Repeat in continuous motion without hesitation. Relax all your muscles that are not pushing your shoulders forward by pressing the pad to move it through space. Keep your breathing automatic without help from your stomach muscles. (See "Breathing Technique.")

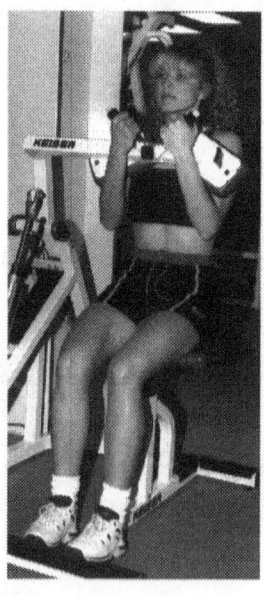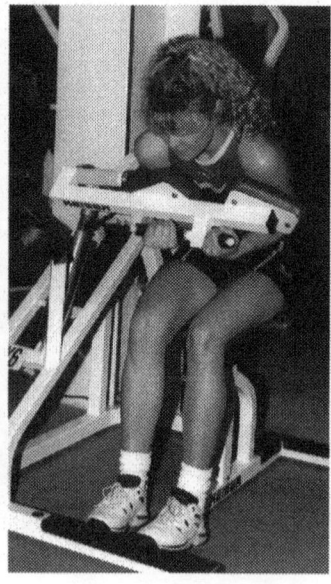

MILITARY PRESS

Sit with your back fully resting on the pad and your spine slightly arched forward by moving your hips back. Hold the handles with an open grip. Press between the stabile endpoints of your shoulders and the movable endpoints of your hands. Press the handles up high without locking your elbows. Return slowly to the starting position. Repeat in continuous motion without hesitation. Relax all your muscles that are not pushing your hands up by pressing the handles to move them through space. Keep your breathing automatic without help from your stomach muscles. (See "Breathing Technique.")

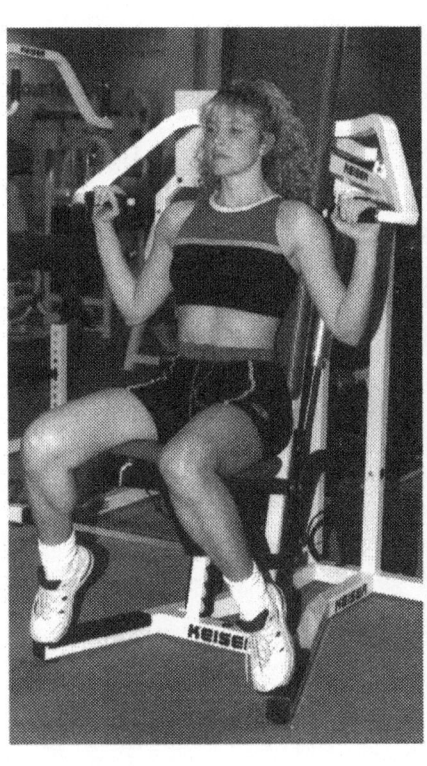 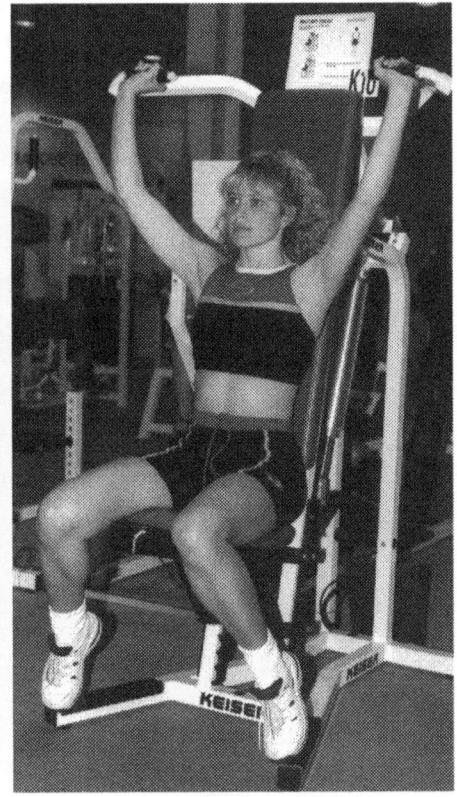

Stretching Technique to Reduce Aches and Increase Range of Motion

Correct stretching is accomplished when you use a technique similar to the one you use for eccentric contraction to lower a weight. For touching your toes, let your torso hang down and concentrate on releasing pressure to let your upper body sink down. The tension of your muscles against the swelling presses fluid out of its pockets. The range of motion increases right from the start of the stretch.

Compressing the swelling with a light, steady pull of the muscles will gradually reduce pressure and let the built-up fluid in the swelled area disperse into a larger area. This is different from pulling hard against the swelling, as when lifting a weight. Pulling hard against the swelling increases the buildup of fluid, as it does in weightlifting. The increase in pressure from heavy pulling to stretch makes the aches more intense and reduces the range of motion. It opposes the main goals of stretching and makes you prone to injuries. Stretching all areas of the body is useful for the relief of tension.

Quadriceps and Shin Stretch

Pull your foot up slowly towards your buttocks until you feel a slight resistance to the stretch. Hold that position and direct your outside muscles (quadriceps and shins) and inside muscles (hamstrings and calves) to stop pressing your foot against your hand. Feel the muscles release fluid and pressure from the pumped areas. Keep moving your foot up as more and more fluid is sent to the rest of the body. Release your foot and repeat with the other leg.

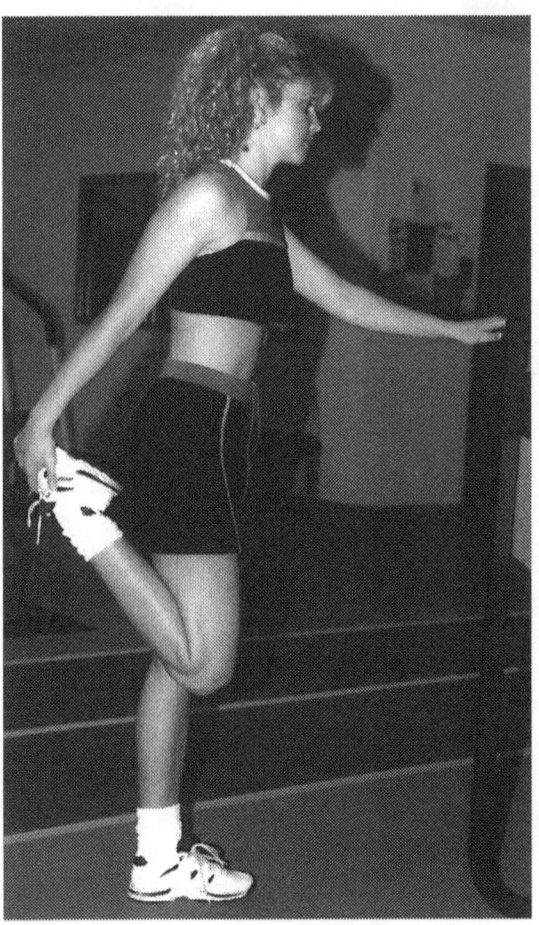

Calf Stretch

Step on the slanted foot pad and hold on to the bar with outstretched arms. Pull your body forward slowly until you feel a slight resistance to the stretch. Hold that position and direct your outside muscles (calves) and inside muscles (shins) to stop pressing your toes against the pads. Feel them release fluid and pressure from the pumped areas. Keep pulling your body forward as more fluid is sent to the rest of the body.

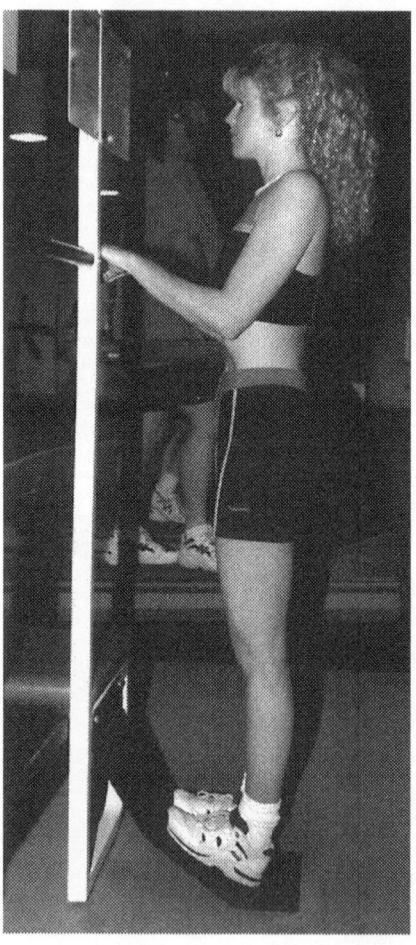

Back, Hams, Glutes, and Calf Stretch

Let your hands drop slowly forward and down while bending at the hip. Reach with your fingertips toward your toes until you feel a slight resistance. Hold that position. Direct the outside muscles of your back, buttocks, thighs, and calfs, and the inside muscles of the stomach and thighs, to stop pushing your shoulders up. Keep lowering your hands as more and more fluid is released to the rest of the body.

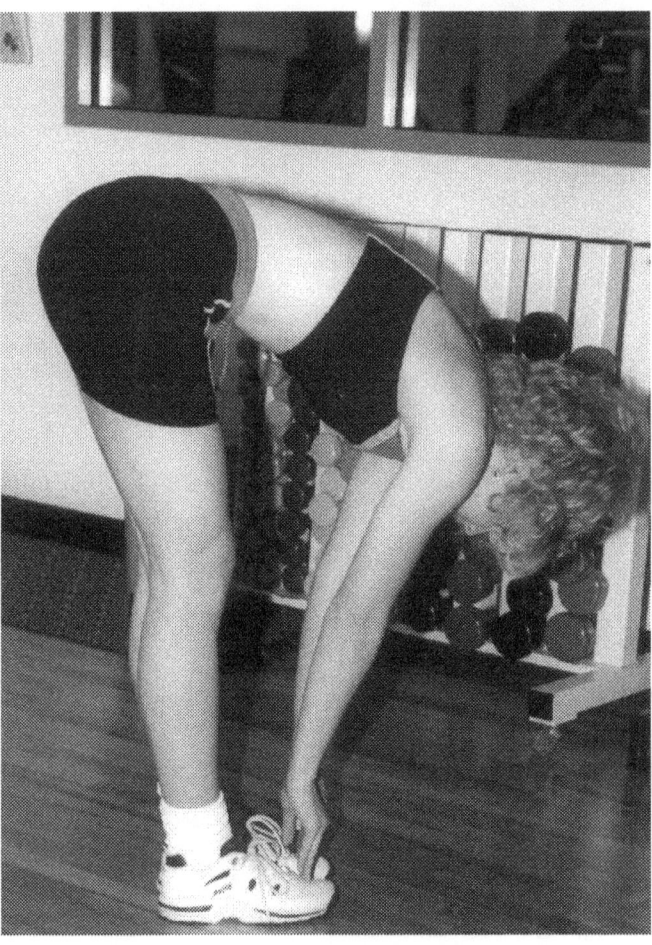

Body and Neck Stretch

Place your hands on your lower back and bend slowly backward at the hip and neck until you feel slight resistance. Hold that position. Tell your outside stomach and your inside neck and lower back muscles to stop pushing your shoulders forward. Let your head and shoulders go a little farther back as fluid is released from the pumped areas.

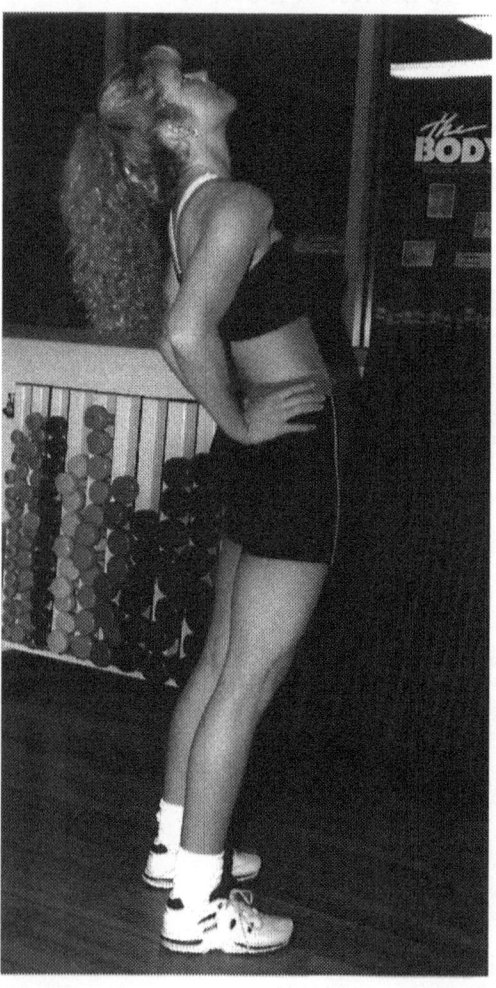

How to Handle Feelings of Numbness, Tension, Aches, and Pain while Running

We all have to face the commonplace discomfort we feel during the times we run. Sometimes it hurts a lot, at other times it's a steady tingling sensation, and then there are the unexpected times when it actually feels light and easy. The feelings can change from moment to moment or last for days. When we look at extraordinary runners, we wonder how they can handle it when they make it look so easy.

Professionals attribute the innocuous aches that runners must live with to tiny tears in the tissues and/or lactic acid buildup due to overuse of the muscles. When we do more exercise than we are accustomed to doing, aches are bound to follow. The day after a harder run, the pain is always more severe. You breathe harder and find it harder to move. Running at your normal pace and distance under increasingly more difficult conditions helps to strengthen your heart and diaphragm and opens up your vascular system.

My anecdotal reasoning is that the aches come from the swelling of pockets that expand in areas of your body where the resilience of the tissues gives way to the pressure from heavy leverage applied against the muscles. I see evidence for my opinion in all the treatments for pain that involve reducing the pressure from swelling. Treatments include ice, massage, stretching, compression, elevation, and blood-thinning drugs. Distributing the swelling to other areas of the body reduces the swelling and gives you a wider range of motion. You also get less pressure against your nerves, which reduces the pain. Nerves become irritated and contribute to pain. Lactic acid and tiny tears in the muscles are widely thought to be the cause.

I once read an article on pain by a well-known sports podiatrist and doctor of preventive medicine. It was about a condition called exertional compartment syndrome (ECS). Runners feel pain from doing too much too soon. Some of the symptoms are tight calves, shin pain, and numbness. ECS is treatable, but it is important to get it diagnosed properly. Exertional Compartment Syndrome is a condition in which lower-leg muscles swell with blood and fluid during and after exercise. The muscle covering (fascia) swells and puts pressure on the nerves inside the muscle compartments. Runners always feel some degree of sensation from pressure against the nerves. The symptoms range from a dull ache to sharp pain. It is hard to know whether it requires medical attention or just the usual home treatments of rest, ice, compression, and elevation. It is best to see a sports physician to rule out other problems.

The doctor may order X rays or a bone scan to check for stress fractures. The procedure for testing for ECS involves checking pressure in the muscle compartment both before and after you run. Some remedies are: new running shoes, physical therapy, orthotics, stretching, and soft tissue massage. Severe cases in athletes—anxious to get back into the game—are treated by making a surgical slit in the fascia. That relieves the pressure that causes the pain and numbness.

Oddly enough, in many cases, couch potatoes feel more pain than runners. Their tissues are less resilient and give way during light pressure. But it's a fact of life that everyone has to live with a certain amount of aches and pains. Most people experience it with a feeling of discomfort and pain. Pressure comes from overloading your muscles by doing more of an activity than you are used to doing on a regular basis. The muscles swell and sting. As long as you don't go beyond the tolerance of your tissues, the overload is the way to build yourself up. "No pain, no gain" is what it takes.

I am one of those people who handle pain by getting pleasure from it. In a way, it is similar to an erotic sensation. I know that what I am feeling isn't harmful. In fact, what is going on is actually making me stronger and healthier. When I go for a run and anticipate what I will be feeling, I say to myself, "Bring it on. I can handle it." When walking or running is part of your normal routine of going places, don't be afraid to press the swelling when it is in your legs. Pressing the swelling when you step down pushes the nerves and makes you feel achy. That kind of ache is not harmful. That pressure is healthy and keeps the blood pumping continuously. Stay loose and happy with the sensation.

There is a way to reduce the severity of the regular aching felt by runners. Simply don't react to it by tensing up. When you land and press with your quadriceps against the hip and the ground, totally relax the rest of your muscles that resist movement. Feel the blood rushing through your body all the way up through your head. Feel it as a good sensation, and don't try to cut it back by tensing all of your muscles together. Later on in the run, when you feel the onset of rising pressure from swelling, be determined to keep relaxed and hold on with the extra pressure until you feel you have had enough, to be safe.

Attitudes that depict running as a grueling and torturous activity are not what you should adopt for yourself. Copy the few runners who put a smile on their faces and feel the excitement of being macho through an activity that has so much to offer. Good attitude will add to the benefits you get from the activity.

At times you will make a misstep that strains a muscle, and it makes you lame. Many times continuing to run easily will relieve it almost instantly. The swelling that results gets dispersed that way. Of course you are taking a chance in doing that. The safest way is to stop running and consult with your doctor. Oftentimes if the injury is slight, you will be recommended to exercise lightly. I have had many occasions when I strained a muscle and ran it out with success. But I don't recommend that others take the risky chances that I take.

Many newcomers to running who haven't done much exercise get easily discouraged. They feel that running is too stressful and too hard for them to handle. That feeling is mostly due to the fact they think that they should be able to push themselves to run like an experienced runner. They start out too fast and are surprised to find out they can't do it.

Almost everyone can become a runner if they start out at an easy pace for themselves. They can start out jogging very slowly for a short distance and mix in some walking. The object is to start exercising a couple of days a week at slightly more physical activity than they are accustomed to and to gradually build from there. Running is hard exercise at any speed. You are lifting a heavy weight for many repetitions. At the same time, you are swinging your body with heavy twisting for many repetitions. If you can handle it, running is a quick way to get fit. Whoever said running exercises the lower part of your body and not the upper part evidently didn't know about the continuous body twists.

If you have any doubts about whether the ache is harmless or harmful, it is always best to check with your doctor.

Training Routines

If you don't know the biomechanics of running, you obviously can't test the effectiveness of training methods. Not many runners are inclined to be highly efficient with their motor skills on their own trial-and-error experimentation. Those that are efficient sometimes get bad advice from professionals who learned science backward. Fortunately, elite runners compare what they are told with what they have developed and wind up choosing their own way. They see that it works better for them. The most notable example is Michael Johnson. His short, choppy movements and upright body running style were good biomechanics. His coaches tried to change it in a way that would have made him worse. He wouldn't change, however, because their way made him slower.

Methods that add speed-work and distance in slight increments are bound to work on runners with more efficient biomechanics. It's the principle of overload—doing more than you are used to doing. But if you are overextending your stride, or trying to push back harder at the ground, you won't advance. Look around at most runners and you will see that with all of their training, they don't progress. Many of the other training methods used are questionable and could be dangerous. Being pulled by a car, running with a parachute, pulling a weighted sled, and plyometrics are some of the popular ones. It is worthwhile to train with the methods that add speed and distance in slight quantities at a time. The following are examples of five classic workouts.

Long Run: Once a week running for 1-1/2 to 2-1/2 hours. It builds your aerobic capacity, opening up circulation and respiration channels, and uses fat as a fuel source.

Fartlek Run: You play with speed by alternating distance running with short bursts of speed. This is a good way to get an interval workout and a feel for altering pace.

Tempo Run: Do a 20 to 30 minute run at 20 to 30 seconds slower than your 5 kilometer race pace. It builds your capacity to run at race pace.

Daily Run: Consistently running most days of the week raises your fitness level and keeps it even.

Repeats: Doing 800 meter repeats at your 10 kilometer race pace, with 2 minutes recovery jogging in between each repeat, pushes your coordination and power.

Training Routines

Before the Guided Muscles technique, which is my running technology, there has never been a worthwhile coaching method that has made a person into a better runner. Runners that did improve did so by using a different technology than what the coaches were giving them.

Training methods are the preeminent tools that coaches rely on to improve runners. These methods were the best the establishment could come up with to be recognized as authorities for making runners faster. Obviously making runners into technically proficient competitors would be the ideal starting point before having them run at all. Unfortunately, the methods the coaches learned in school weren't working. As a matter of fact, they were impossible to execute.

A sense of balance is needed to become a fast runner. Some runners have a better sense than others and can improve with a variety of training methods. A good sense of balance allows a runner to speed up with each step and reach a higher speed than runners with a poor sense of balance. With my methods, balance for speed can be learned to allow you to fall and recover faster than you could with just a feel for speed. Technically, you are always in balance when you are stabilized in your motion.

Preparing for a race as a beginner can be daunting and disappointing if you think of it as a test of how much pain you can take. You must realize that you are not racing anyone but yourself. If you make the same mistake most beginners make and sprint out fast at the start, you will be running with much discomfort soon after you start. Use your training sessions to give you an idea of how you should pace yourself. To make it a worthwhile race, try a little faster than your usual training pace and see what happens.

Beginner Training

This typical training routine for beginner runners is not something I am qualified to recommend for anyone to follow. The basic understanding of beginning an exercise program with only slightly more vigorous activity than you are normally accustomed to doing makes sense to me. This chart is only meant to familiarize you with the type of schedules that are being devised for runners who like to follow a routine. Consistent training maintains a steady level of fitness. When you have periods in which you don't train for a while, your fitness level drops, and it becomes harder to run. When you return to running at your previous pace, it will be harder to do. If you do not slow your pace for a while, you will over-train. I stopped entering races because they are inconvenient for me. I like getting down to the health club and working out to stay in good physical shape.

Beginner Runner 6-Week
Training Schedule for 5k Race

WEEK	SUN.	MON.	TUES.	WED.	THUR.	FRI.	SAT.	TOTAL
	Miles	Miles	Miles	Miles	Miles	Miles	Miles	Miles
1	1.5	Rest	1.5	Rest	1.5	1	Rest	5
2	2	Rest	2	Rest	1.5	1	Rest	6.5
3	2.5	Rest	2.5	Rest	2	1.5	Rest	8.5
4	3	Rest	3	Rest	2.5	2	Rest	11
5	3.5	1.5	2.5	Rest	2.5	1.5	Rest	13
6 Taper	Rest	3.5	1.5	Rest	1.5	Rest	RACE	9.6

Intermediate Training

This typical training routine for intermediate runners is not something I am qualified to recommend for anyone to follow. The basic understanding of improving speed by including short periods of slightly faster running than in typical distance training makes sense to me. Keep in mind that the faster you run makes you more prone to injuries.

Intermediate Runner 6 Week
Training Schedule for 5k Race

WEEK	SUN.	MON.	TUES.	WED.	THUR.	FRI.	SAT.	TOTAL
	Intervals	Miles	Hills	Training	Miles	Miles	Training	
	Meters	Easy	Minutes		Easy	Easy		
1	6X400	3	6	0	3	5	0	22
2	2x800	3	6	0	3	5	0	22
	2x400							
	2x200							
3	2x800	3	7	0	3	6	0	24
	2x400							
	4x200							
4	3x800	3	7	0	3	6	0	25
	2x400							
	2x200							
5	2X800	3	7	0	3	7	0	28
	4X400							
	4X200							
6 Taper	4X400	3	0	3X200	1	0	RACE	
	4X200			3X150				
				6X100				

Advanced Training

This typical training routine for advanced runners is not something I am qualified to recommend for anyone to follow. The basic understanding of improving speed by including short periods of slightly faster running in your distance training makes sense to me. Adding distance and speed is a tough routine to follow. You must be in excellent shape to do it.

Advanced Runner 6 Week
Training Schedule for 5k Race

WEEK	SUN.	MON.	TUES.	WED.	THUR.	FRI.	SAT.	TOTAL
	Intervals	Miles	Intervals	Training	Miles	Miles	Training	
	Meters	Easy	Meters		Easy	Easy		
1	1X1200	5	2x800	0	5	8	0	33
	2X800		2x400					
	4X100		4x200					
2	10x300	5	2x1200	0	5	8	0	33
	4x100		1x800					
			2x400					
			4x200					
3	2x1200	5	2x800	0	5	9	0	34
	2x800		4x400					
	2x400		4x200					
	4x400							
4	3x800	5	3x800	0	5	9	0	35
	4x100		3x400					
			3x200					
			2x100					
5	2x1200	5	4x400	0	5	9	0	36
	2x800		4x300					
	2x400		4x200					
	2x200		4x100					
6 Taper	2x400	3	4X200	0	2	1	RACE	
	2x300		4X100					
	2x200							
	6x100							

Walking—Just Undo It

Walking is different from running by only one feature: in walking both feet are never in the air together. Otherwise, walking can be seen as running. It uses the same running technology of moving by the power of gravity. If you are not falling forward, you are not able to walk.

There is a balance in all movement that stabilizes you. The technology for both walking and running starts with positioning your foot to set you off balance when you are standing in place. With your weight ahead of the supporting foot, gravity makes you fall forward.

The walking movement doesn't look like a falling motion because both feet are on the ground—one in back and one in front. Your back foot lifts your body by your leg rising up on your toe. During the lift, your body is falling forward off your back foot until it creates enough speed to pass your forward foot. When your body passes your forward foot, the falling process starts again.

The important part of walking that often gets it overlooked as a gravity-powered activity is what happens in the lift. When your back foot extends to put more pressure against your upper body, your front leg loses the pressure to support your body. Even though both feet are on the ground, only the back foot is supporting your body. Since your weight is ahead of the back foot, your body falls ahead of the back foot as it does in running.

The fact that the spread of the feet is slower in walking means that there is enough time to bring the raised foot forward to catch your body before it falls too low and prevents the return of your foot going forward. When you increase your walking speed beyond your ability to return the foot forward, your whole body tenses up and holds you back in an attempt to keep you from falling. You have the ability to go faster at that point, but only if you take to the air with both feet to give your-self more time to exchange your feet. When you do that, you can relax again because your sense of balance will feel comfortable again.

Our sense of balance is not developed equally in individuals. When we sense that we will be off balance traveling at a certain speed, we tense up. At a fast walking speed, our feet are forced to spread farther apart. Your supporting leg is dragged farther back. When the speed gets too fast for walking, your feet cannot return fast enough to balance the fall in time. At that point, both feet must take to the air together for more air time. This gives you the extra time you needed to exchange your feet, allowing you to move faster. In all categories of self-transport—walking, jogging, running, and sprinting—the same technology applies. The more you drop your feet towards the rear, the faster you will go.

Walking is easiest and healthiest when you coordinate your whole body to react to the force of gravity with the least muscular force needed. When you apply extra force above and beyond what is required for the speed at which you are moving, the extra work is caused only by the things that you are doing to resist the action.

The walking process is essentially the same as running, and as such utilizes the same body twist to exchange the feet in time to stay in bal-ance. You know from Newton's Third Law, "for every action there is an equal and opposite reaction." Well, the equal and opposite reaction of shooting the foot forward is shooting the hip back. Shooting the hip back is not something we want to happen, because when both ends move (your foot and hip), power is lessened at both ends. What we've learned to do by feeling is to drive your shoulder forward on the oppo-site side of your foot that is moving forward. The equal and opposite action of that movement of shooting your shoulder forward is shooting your hip forward. By shooting your hip back and forward from oppo-site sides, your hip is locked and won't rotate. There we have an immovable platform to shoot the leg forward without loss of power.

Your arm shooting forward ahead of your shoulder adds power to shoot your hip forward. Positioning your arms straight down or bent at an approximate 90-degree angle for walking is all a matter of what feels most comfortable. Keeping your arms down is more relaxing for walking.

The best posture for walking is the same as for every upright stance you take. The objective is to put as little muscle effort as you can into keeping the body from collapsing. First you must realize that the spine is not located in the center of the chest, so the chest is not balanced on the spine when the spine is erect. The weight of the chest and the head ahead of the spine places stress on the muscles to stop the spine from being pulled down. To correct the posture, put a slight arch in your lower back to bring the hip forward and the chest back. That way the chest is centered on the spine. A slight arch in the neck balances the head on the spine.

A very common mistaken impression people have is that tilting the upper body shifts their balance to make them run faster. That impression has been proven wrong, and yet many professionals still adhere to it. Record-breaking sprints have been made with an upright posture. This proves that the angle of the upper body is not the balance shift for producing speed. After all, can't you stand still when your upper body is slanted forward? You can even run backward with your upper body tilted forward. When you tilt your upper body forward while standing still, your body is automatically shifted to center you for standing still. The same thing happens when you are walking. Your body is automatically shifted to keep you moving at the same pace, no matter how much you tilt your upper body. The only thing that will increase speed for you is when you drop your feet more to the rear of your weight. This holds true for a slanted or upright posture.

Landing technique is important for walking even though it is not as hard on the joints as running. Touching the ground softly with your toe slightly raised, and then pressing with the full weight of the body on a flat foot is best. The three pads of your foot, one behind the arch and two in front of it, spread the pressure across a wide surface. The wider surface cushions the pressure better.

Walking and running are the ideal exercises for pumping blood through the entire body. The weight of your body coming down hard on your foot sends pooled blood flowing from the farthest extremity up to your heart and the other extremities. There are many health benefits to having a substantial amount of blood saturating the body and bringing nutrients to more parts of the body. Knowing and using the right technology for moving with a relaxed body opens the circulatory channels wider.

Pointing your foot straight ahead keeps your joints rolling in a smooth, centered path. This protects them from rubbing the joints and nerves in a way that causes wear and pain. Landing with the foot pointed to the side twists your muscles and injures them.

Keeping the knee slightly bent at landing absorbs the weight better. Many people, especially heavyset individuals, experience a backward snap of the knee when their knee is straight at landing. It damages the muscles around the joint.

Overstriding and dropping the foot back before landing bring the foot down on the ground and the ground moving at the same speed, so there is no pressure front and back.

A very short stride length gives you the ability to pick up phenomenal speed with each step, but it is not required for walking. A medium stride length is more comfortable and less stressful.

A shorter reach ahead of the body gives you a faster pace than a long reach. Dropping the foot five inches ahead of the body is faster than dropping the foot six inches ahead of the body. Gravity pulls you harder when your weight is more to the front in your stride.

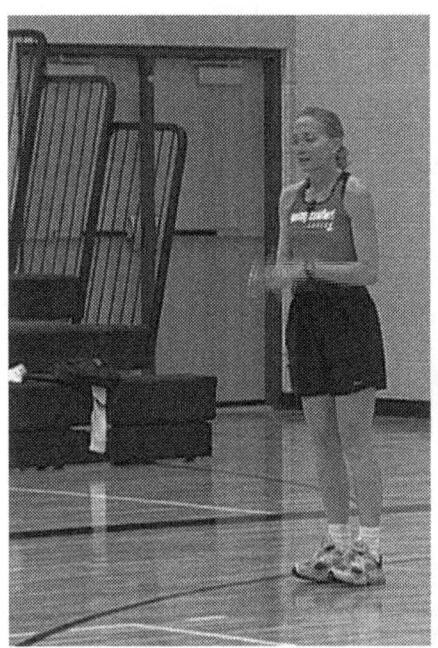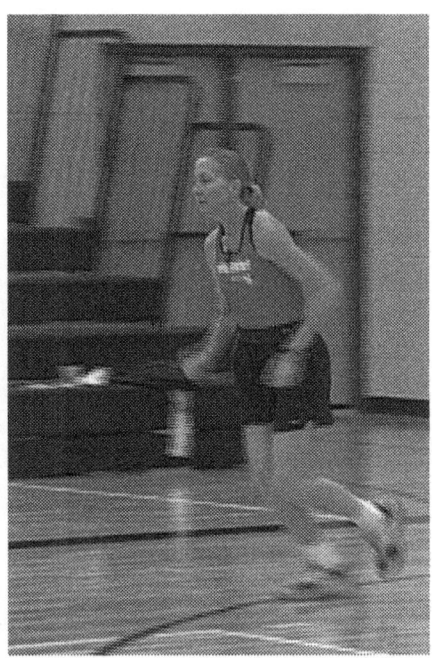

The only way that you can move your body forward is by positioning your feet so that your weight is ahead of them. With the first step, when you lift your toes it removes the front support of your body and you fall forward. You do not use any muscles to try to push, because it is impossible to do while your lower leg is being pressed forward to lift. Your leg rolls forward on the foot as your body drags the top of your leg forward.

Your first step is always very slow and can be stopped by reaching far ahead or sped up by dropping the feet to the rear of the body. Many people can't picture how to drop their feet to the rear of their body. It's done by letting your body fall far ahead of the supporting foot and dropping the other foot just a little ahead of the supporting foot. Keeping your feet dropping to the rear of your body increases speed with each step. You eliminate the slowdown phase of the stride. At an even pace, your foot drops slightly ahead of the body. A walker increases speed with each step for two or three strides, while a sprinter takes many more steps by dropping his feet behind his body.

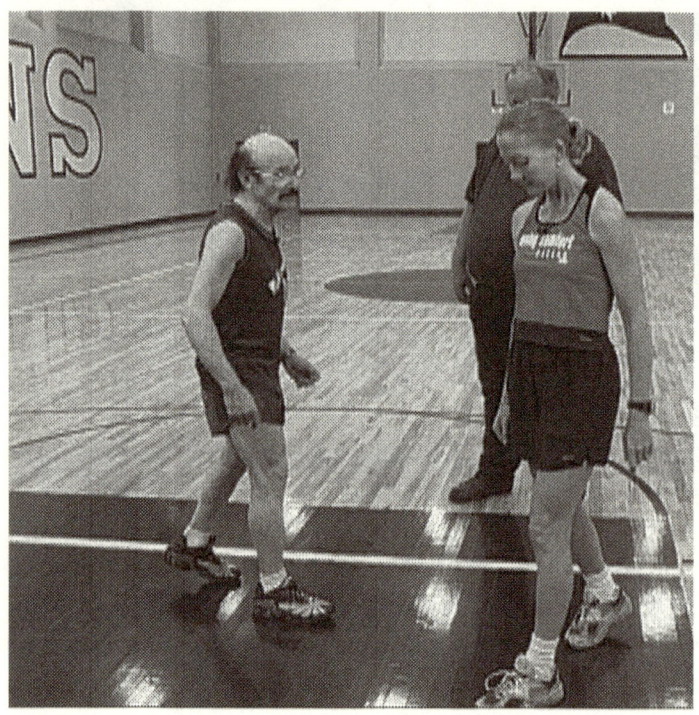

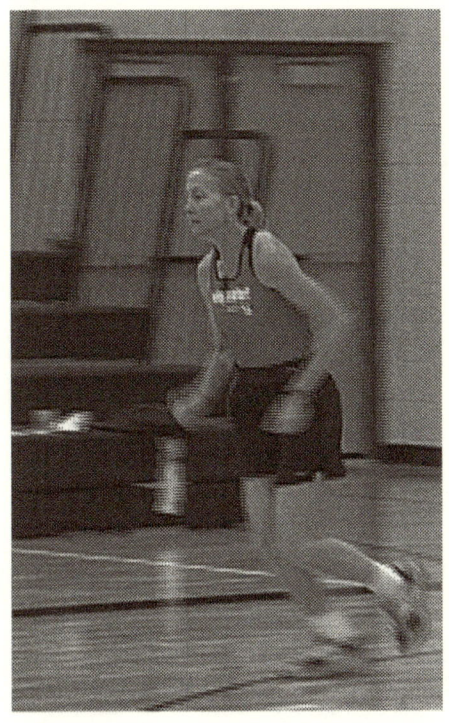

Your leg does not push your body forward in this position either. Raising your body with your back leg takes the weight off of your front foot. Your weight being on your back foot and out in front of it gets pulled forward by gravity. Your front foot appears to be landing farther ahead than it actually is. It has been made to overstride and is falling back while your body is moving forward. By the time your front foot is fully pressed to the ground, your foot is close to the center of your body. The forward reach is actually short.

A difficult thing for people to visualize is that tilting their upper body forward is not the type of lean that creates movement. Your sense of balance will keep you at the same pace when your body is erect as when it is tilted forward. A perfect example is that when standing still, tilting your upper body forward doesn't make you fall forward. You remain standing in place, unless you raise your toes to knock you off balance. An erect body is easier on your back muscles.

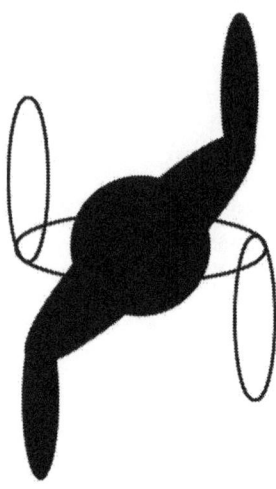

The body-twist part of the running and walking process is a major part of the effort. Contrary to popular belief, the upper body gets a lot of exercise from the power needed to exchange the feet using a body twist. Of course, less overall power is needed when you are moving slowly. Many walkers twist their bodies hard to exchange the feet and arms. They do it to get a more intense workout.

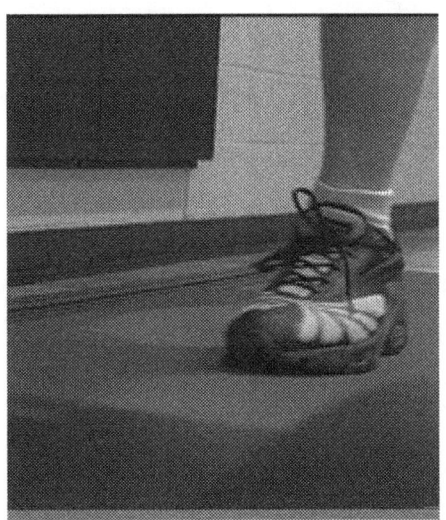

Overstriding a little and then dropping your foot back and down while it is still in the air prepares you for a soft landing. Instead of locking your knee and waiting for your body to drop, lower your foot to touch the ground lightly. The backward drop is natural for many people and animals, but not in a safe way. They use backward pressure by hitting back at the ground faster than the ground is moving away. They do that to try to push them forward. Instead of pushing them forward, it can cause hamstring injury. You cannot pull your supporting leg back once your foot touches down, because it is pushing forward to support and lift your body. The backward drop should match the speed of the ground moving back. This way it is not adding impact in a forward or backward direction. Touch the ground lightly with your toe slightly raised, then press fully with your foot flat to support your body. The flat landing spreads the pressure across a larger area. Make sure your foot is pointing straight ahead so the joints will be seated properly.

Racewalking—Just Undo It

The distinguishing elements in racewalking technology are the tilting of the hips from side to side and the arms swinging from side to side. The tilting of the hips does not get more speed out of gravity. Anything that you can also do slowly is not the gravity technology for speed. The only thing that gets more speed out of gravity is when you drop your feet more to the rear than what you are doing. You can't go slower that way, or stay at the same pace.

Tilting your hip sideways is used to bring your raised foot forward while skimming along close to the ground. By keeping your forward-swinging foot low, there can be a quicker weight transfer from one foot to the other. That allows both of your feet to be in contact with the ground for a split second to qualify as walking. The rules are that the front foot must touch the ground before the back foot leaves the ground, and the leg must be straight as the body passes it.

Elite racewalkers can walk much faster than the average runner. The quicker transfer of the weight allows them to drop their feet more to the rear than the walkers who don't tilt their hips. It still takes a lot of energy to walk at competitive racewalking speed. You need to train hard and develop good balance for speed.

Racewalking is a good alternative to running for people who can't be persuaded to run for fear of injuring themselves. When done smoothly, you can get the health benefits of running without some of the trauma.

Racewalkers keep their toe high to distinguish the motion from running. All of the running technology applies to racewalking as well. As I mentioned before, walking, racewalking, jogging, running, and sprinting are all powered by gravity in the same way. Dropping your feet to the rear puts you in balance for forward motion. Gravity will not allow anybody to stand still unless his or her weight is centered over his or her feet. When the weight is centered, no muscles can push it forward. There is no way to begin moving forward except to reposition your feet or foot to the rear.

Smooth running techniques are vital to keep racewalking safe and fast. Over-striding and dropping your foot back before touching down smoothes your landing. This puts no backward or forward pressure against the ground. You just stand neutral on the ground, while you roll forward on the ankle and toe.

Reaching down while returning your foot toward the rear has the effect of touching the ground softly, before pressing down fully with the full weight of your body. This prohibits a jolting collision with the ground.

The touch of your foot on the ground can't be done without a slight slowdown because of the forward reach of your leg. That slowdown immediately changes to a speedup when your leg passes a vertical position and your body falls forward. During the speedup you should feel your leg being dragged back by the ground. All effort to pull your leg back should be avoided.

Exchanging your feet in time to keep you in balance with the speed is powered by a body twist. In a twist the opposite ends turn in opposite directions while the center doesn't rotate. Making your hip the center of your body twist locks your hip to keep it from rotating. This makes the hip an immovable platform to send your left foot and right shoulder forward, and vice versa. Your foot shooting forward pushes your hip back and your shoulder shooting forward pushes your hip forward. The pushes at the hip from opposite sides lock the hip sideways. The swinging of the arms assists in the upper body twist.

Your feet should always be pointing forward so that the joints can roll centered in their sockets. If your hip turns, your foot will also turn, so lock your hip.

Training to balance yourself for altering your speed as fast as you can is best done by noticing how high your feet get flipped by the speed while you are twisting your hardest to keep them down.

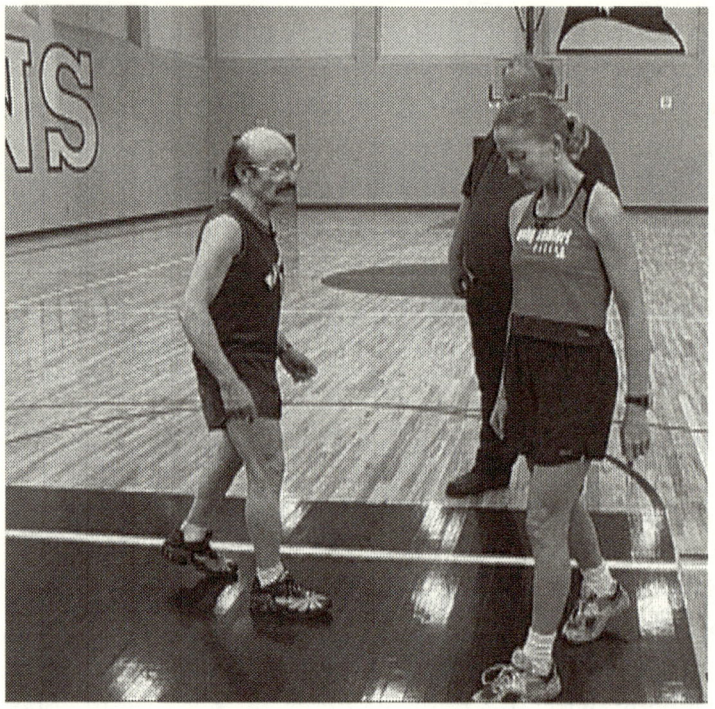

Walking has all of the same technology as running. If your intention is to limit your speed, you can start off with a longer stride and never reach a fast speed that requires both feet to be in the air together. The only reason you toss yourself up higher to run is to allow more time to exchange your feet. Your feet are spread farther apart by increased speed. By moving faster, your leg must travel a farther distance back and up, and then to return. With racewalking, the intention is to go as fast as you can and still have one foot touching the ground before the other one leaves the ground. Another rule that separates racewalking from running is that in racewalking the supporting leg is kept straight as the body travels over it. That prevents you from jumping up. The racewalking technique is to come forward with your heel skimming very close to the ground. This allows the touch-down and liftoff to be made faster. Your hip is tilted down to keep your heel very low to the ground.

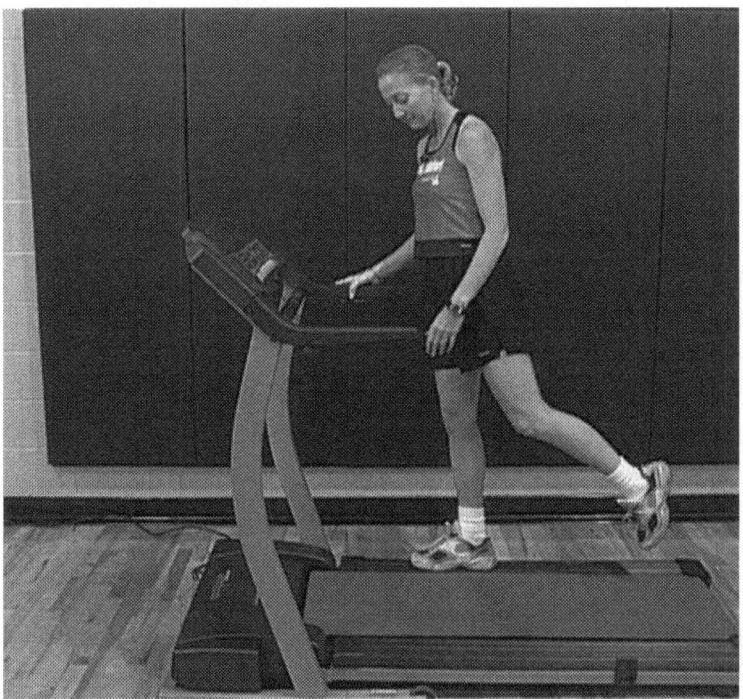

Racewalking can't reach anywhere near the speed of sprinting, but a good racewalker goes faster than most distance runners. The body twist that powers the exchange of the feet is different from the running technique. The rotation of the upper body is greater for racewalking, to help with the tilting of the hip. The foot is not flipped back and up as high, because the speed isn't as fast as that of a top runner.

Treadmill Running or Walking

Training on a treadmill rather than on the road or a track is very popular for many good reasons.

* The surface is softer to run on.
* You can measure the speed, distance, and hills better.
* You can run alongside someone at a different pace.
* You can watch TV or listen to the radio or CDs.
* You are protected from the weather elements.
* You are safer from predators.
* You can stop if you need to, without having to travel back.
* You don't have to carry water or medical supplies.
* You don't have to concentrate on maintaining your speed.
* You can do it at home and not miss any calls or deliveries.
* You can analyze your form in a mirror or have a professional do it.
* It's a good way to teach people how to run.

People are under the impression that you can push yourself forward to run. That is why they don't see it as amazing that they can run on a treadmill at all. The first time someone starts to walk or run on a treadmill they are off balance and have to make adjustments to stay aligned with the frame while their feet are being dragged back.

The adjustment they make is not based on how hard they push; the push is not possible to do. They automatically adjust their balance for the speed to a precise landing spot ahead of their body, which will allow them to match their falling speed to the speed of the belt. It is all done by feel, without knowing the technology of what powers the running movement. To run at the speed of the belt, you cannot alter the angle of the landing leg at which you are balanced. If you do, you will no longer match the speed of the belt. Drop your feet to the rear of that balanced landing spot and you will pick up speed and hit the front of the treadmill. Drop your feet more to the front of the balanced landing spot and you will lose speed and fall off the back of the treadmill.

Changing your pace is not done by adjusting your balance when you are holding on to the treadmill frame. The frame won't let you alter your position for gravity to pull you forward. Holding on to the frame stops your body from traveling back with the belt. Your supporting leg gets pulled back at the speed of the belt no matter what angle it lands at. This kind of running is quite different than the normal way of being powered by gravity. Holding on to the treadmill frame is not as healthy as natural running. The upper body is held stiff and doesn't get the extra circulation by swinging the shoulders and arms. Instead of holding on to the sensor on the frame that monitors your heart rate, you can wear a separate device.

Many runners hold on to the frame when they set their treadmill on an incline. Doing so does more damage than running on a level platform while holding on. The stress on the upper body is greater on an incline.

When you run normally on an incline, gravity pulls forward and down while you jump higher to glide level with the ground. The higher jump works harder against gravity and the landing is softer than when you run on level terrain. There are special treadmills that you can tilt lower in front to let you run downhill. Gravity powers you down and forward downhill while you lower your body to glide level with the ground. The landing angle slows you more to match the faster speedup from gravity. Downhill running is harder than running on level terrain.

All of the running technology applies to treadmills as well. As I mentioned before, walking, racewalking, jogging, running, and sprinting are all powered by gravity in the same way. Dropping your feet to the rear puts you in balance for forward motion. Gravity will not allow anybody to stand still unless their weight is centered over their feet or a foot. When the weight is centered, no muscles can push it forward.

There is no way to get moving forward other than to reposition your feet or foot to the rear.

Smooth running techniques are vital to keep treadmill running safe and fast. Overstriding and dropping your foot back before touching down smoothes the landing; it avoids putting backward or forward pressure against the ground. You just stand neutral on the ground, while you roll forward on your ankle and toe.

Reaching down while returning your foot toward the rear has the effect of touching the ground softly, before pressing down fully with the full weight of your body. This prohibits a jolting collision with the ground.

The touch of your foot on the ground can't be done without a slight slowdown because of the forward reach of your leg. The slowdown immediately changes to a speedup when your leg passes a vertical position and your body falls forward. During the speedup you should feel your leg being dragged back by the ground. All effort to pull the leg back should be avoided.

Exchanging your feet in time to keep you in balance with the speed is powered by a body twist. In a twist, the opposite ends turn in opposite directions while the center doesn't rotate. Making your hip the center of your body twist locks your hip to keep it from rotating. That makes your hip an immovable platform from which to send your left foot and right shoulder forward, and vice versa. Your foot shooting forward pushes your hip back, and your shoulder shooting forward pushes your hip forward. The pushes at the hip from opposite sides lock the hip sideways. The swinging of the arms assists in the upper body twist.

Your feet should always be pointing forward so that the joints can roll centered in their sockets. If your hips turn, your feet will also turn, so lock your hip.

Training to balance yourself for altering your speed as fast as you can is best done by noticing how high your feet get flipped by the speed while you are twisting your hardest to keep them down.

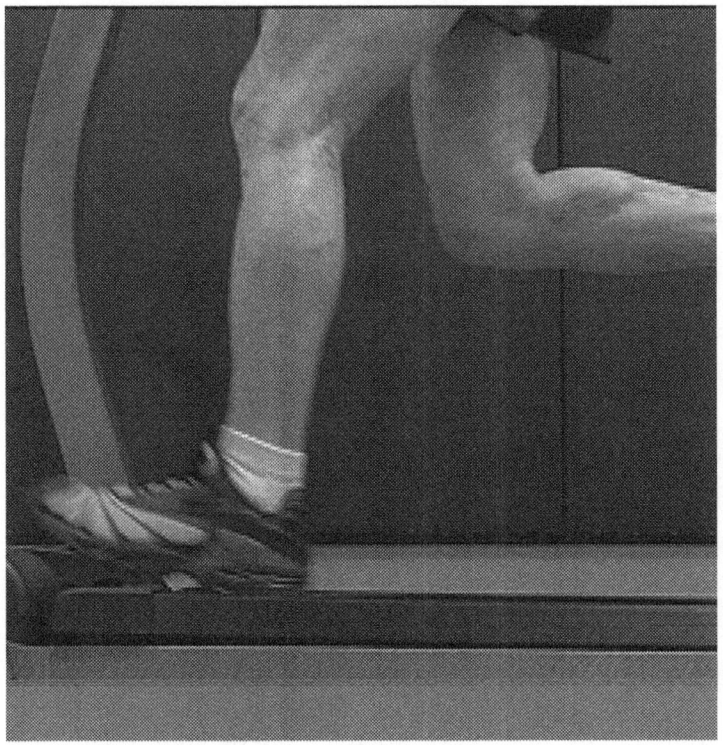

The belt is moving back rapidly. It is going to the rear of the runner just as fast as the stationary ground moves to the rear of the runner going at the same pace. You can now see that treadmill running uses the same physics and technology as road running. The treadmill is a perfect place to test my running techniques using gravity. I was able to see that changing the reach for the landing changed the speed of the run. In the reach shown above, the foot has not yet landed. It is being brought back to a speed that matches the backward speed of the belt. That serves two purposes: The foot doesn't impact against the belt and doesn't produce as much of a kickback against the speed. This is yet another one of my ways to make running easier on the joints.

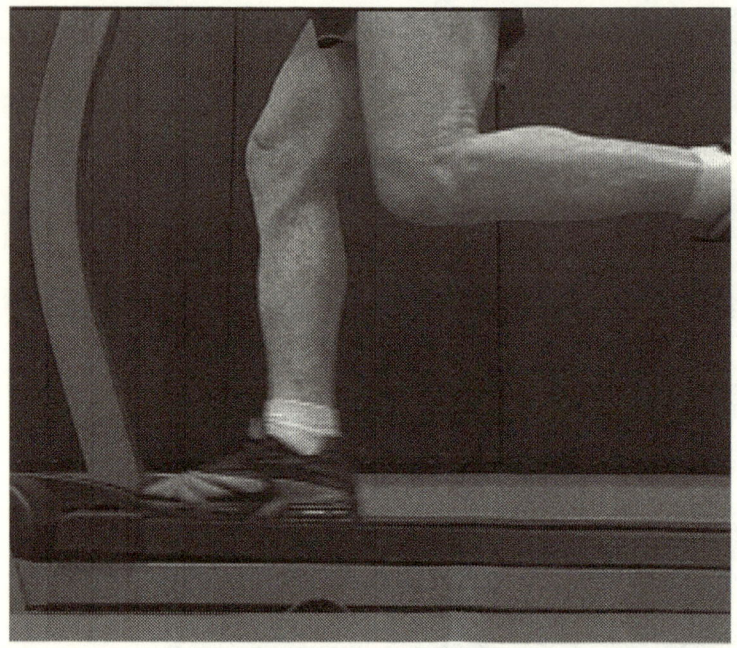

When your foot moves back from the over-stride, it touches down with your body's full weight at a short reach ahead of your body. The shorter you make the reach, the faster gravity propels you. The more you drop your foot to the rear, the faster you will be running. The more you drop your foot to the front, the slower you will be running. The landing spot is the only thing that sets you off balance while standing still and makes you fall forward at varying speeds.

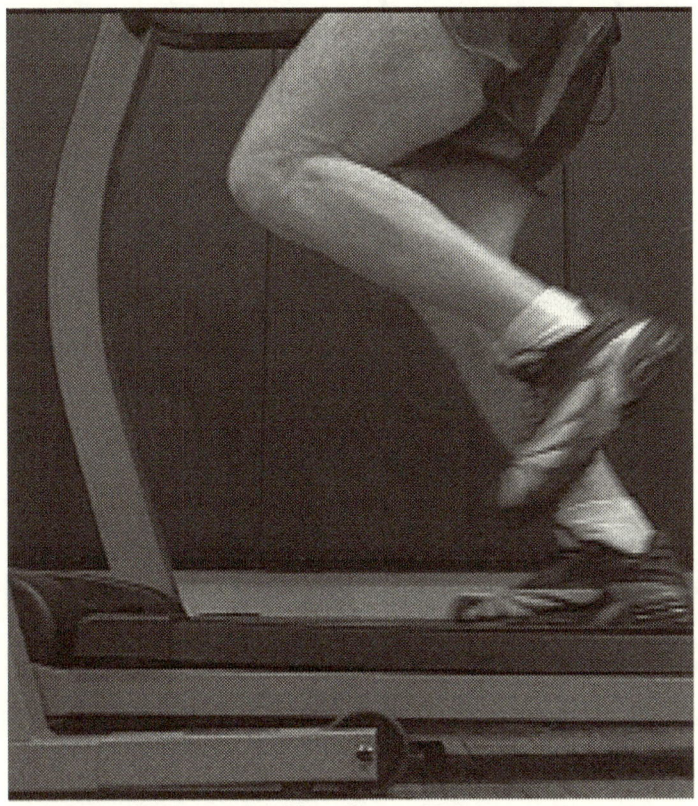

The forward knee drive taught by other instructors is a poor way to describe the power needed to return the foot to a forward reach. The emphasis needs to be on driving the whole leg forward. Leaving the lower leg high while you drive just the knee forward will delay the return of the foot. Notice again that the supporting foot is moving back with the belt while rolling at the ankle. The leg rolls forward just like a vaulting pole. When you just stand still and let gravity pull you, the feeling is much easier than if you try to push back. Feel the ground pulling your foot back while you are just standing still; after all, you are standing still when trying to push or not trying to push. Either way, it's your body that is moving forward.

Clarifying and Proving the Technology

Many people cannot follow any instruction manual no matter how simple the technology or how well it is presented. The technology in this book is very simple to grasp. It is based on gravity. Who can't predict what gravity will do? The following examples will clarify and prove how gravity is the universal driving force for running.

The leg acts like a vaulting pole that relies on momentum and gravity to vault the body forward. The leg is at a backward slant when it hits the ground and at a forward slant when it leaves the ground. That is exactly what a vaulting pole does for a forward vault, which is level with the ground. Running technology, from walking to sprinting, uses the vaulting action to send the body forward. The knee is locked by the quadriceps muscles at landing and straightens the leg along with the calf muscles to extend the foot for lifting the body. There is no backward push in a vault. The bottom of the leg rolls when the top is gliding forward.

The body cannot start moving from a balanced position for standing still when the feet are together. The forward movement can only be started by lifting the toe. The front support is no longer there so gravity sends the body gliding forward.

The body cannot move when its weight is equally distributed between the two legs while one is forward and the other is back. The only way you can get your body moving forward from that position is to lift up with your back leg. Lifting up with your back leg takes the weight of your body off of the front leg and places it on the back leg. Your body, being ahead of the back foot, falls forward and passes the front foot. This starts the cycle of the body being vaulted from one leg to the other.

Rock back and forth, lifting the toes and then the heels. When you were standing still, your weight was centered between your heels and your toes. By lifting the front support (the toes), you have shifted the supporting legs behind the weight. The weight of your body, being ahead of the supporting heels, falls forward because it is pulled by the force of gravity. When the toes come down and the heels lift up, the legs are shifted ahead of the weight and the body falls back. This demonstrates how the body runs without a push by the legs. The legs roll on the ankle and the toe while the top of the leg is gliding forward.

Place your hands against a wall, with your arms shoulder-high and fully extended, and with your body slightly ahead of your feet. Notice that the weight of your body is pushing you lightly against the wall. Try to push back against the ground and you will see that you cannot push any harder against the wall than the power of gravity. Gravity is the only power that can pull you forward for running.

Now place your hands against the wall, with your arms shoulder-high and the arms fully extended, and with your feet further back from the wall. Notice that the weight of the body is pushing you much harder against the wall. Try to push back against the ground and you will find that you cannot push any harder against the wall than the power of gravity. Gravity is the only power that pulls you forward—not the muscles pushing.

Place your hands against a wall, with your arms shoulder-high and the arms fully extended, and with the feet far back from the wall. Jump up and notice that the jump didn't push your body any harder against the wall. The legs were pushing down and forward to jump straight up. During running the legs push the body straight up. Only the falling of the body by gravity pulling you is what makes you fall forward. The jump allows you to glide level with the ground. Notice also that the front muscles across the knee push down and forward to jump. Pulling the back muscles back and up is impossible to do while running.

Run alongside a partner for about forty yards while each of you is using an opposite technique. One person pushes back against the ground for a hard push forward (or tries to do it) and leaps forward as far as he can. The other person twists his body as hard as he can to keep his stride as short as possible. At the same time he should be dropping his feet as far toward the rear as he can. Change techniques with the other partner and try it again. This will prove that only gravity can produce the speed. Trying to push makes you work harder and accomplish less.

Many runners won't easily give up their belief that the body is pushed forward by muscles. Some can't cope with the fact that they weren't the masterful runners they thought they were. The professionals find it especially hard to swallow. I can appreciate how Galileo felt when he was trying to convince the experts.

These examples are perfect for changing the minds of all those who doubt that the force of gravity pulls you forward and not the muscles pushing.

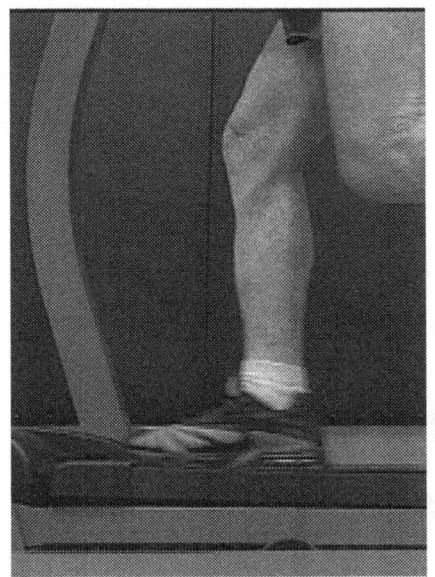
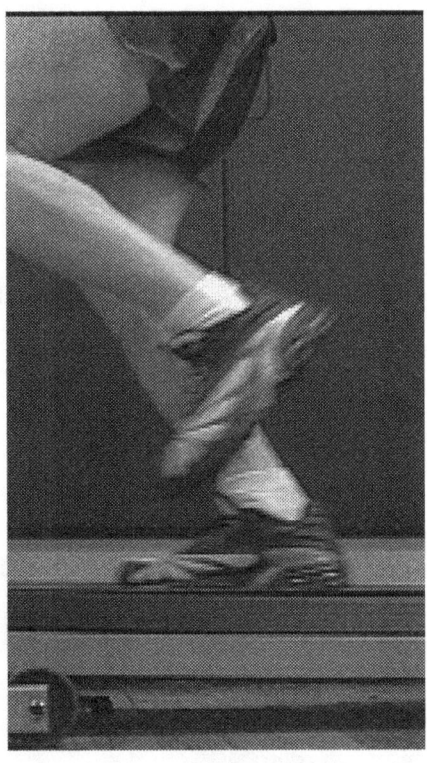

The supporting leg acts as if it is a vaulting pole. The top of the leg moves from behind the foot to in front of it. With a flat foot landing, the ankle rolls forward on the socket of the foot. The knee is locked in a bent position, making the leg one solid unit, just like a pole. Once the foot is placed ahead of the body, the pace is set and cannot be changed. Momentum carries the top of the leg to a vertical position, and then gravity picks up the speed from there. The air time and the landing ahead of the body are the slowdown phase. It is matched by the pickup phase to level the pace. After you plant the foot, there is no action you can take with your upper body or your legs to alter the pace for the rest of the stride. Tilting your upper body does nothing for speed. You can run backward with the upper body tilted forward. Maintaining a consistent vertical position of your upper body is the easiest on your back muscles. You can reach ahead of the weight equally with a vertical body as with a tilted one.

When the top of the leg falls ahead of the foot and the ground, the foot is dragged back by the ground. After the landing you should feel your foot being pulled back, while your leg is not pushing your foot back or forward. Your leg should be bent to absorb the landing and in a position to lift your body with the help of the heel lift. The toss-up does not propel the body forward. Falling propels the body forward, while lifting the body keeps it level with the ground. Pushing off from the toe does not add speed. You need to raise your body just enough to glide level with the ground. Jumping any higher for a long stride will slow you down. Dropping the foot five inches ahead of the weight is faster running than dropping it six inches ahead.

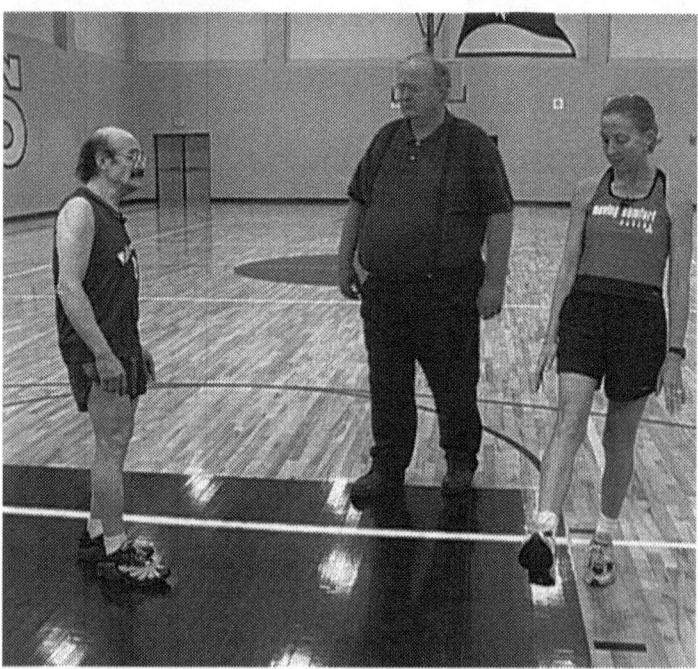

It is said that walking is as simple as putting one foot in front of the other, but doing so isn't what makes you go forward. You can do it and stand still, or even fall backward. Anything you can do while standing still is not a power move for running. You can also try to push back as hard as you can and stand still when your weight is centered between your heel and your toe. Lifting your toe without pushing back will send you forward in the only way that is possible for it to be done—by having gravity pulling you.

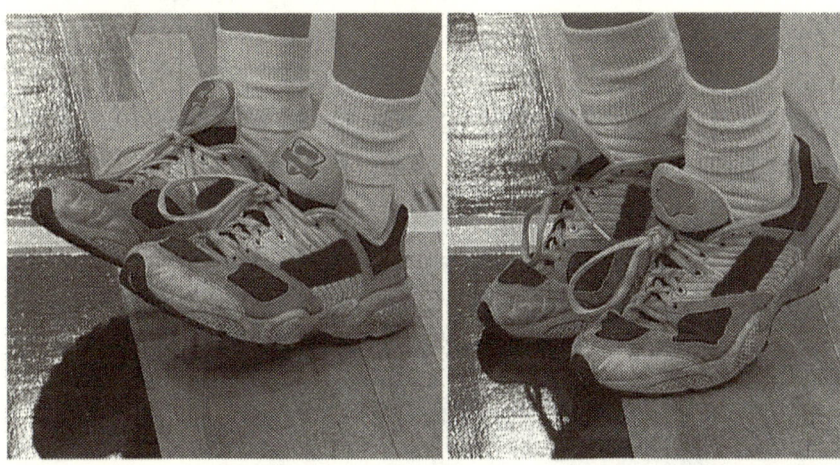

Keep your weight centered between your heel and your toes. Lift your toes to remove the front support and your weight is shifted in front of its support at the heels. You can now predict that you will be falling forward without a push by muscles. Gravity is the obvious force that is moving you forward. It is the only force that can do it for walking and running. The planet with the heaviest pull of gravity is where you can run the fastest. You are an expert in what gravity will do, so this is easy to understand. Why researchers missed seeing it is a mystery.

Keep your weight centered between your heels and your toes. Lift your heels to remove the back support and your weight is shifted in back of its support at the toes. Now you are falling back. You can see that happening without trying it. You cannot increase the speed of rocking back and forth, no matter how hard you try to push back at the ground. You cannot increase the force of rocking forward by pushing back at the ground. Surprisingly, you can increase the force to rock backward by adding a forward push against the ground. You always push forward in both directions to support and lift your body, so that is the only direction your muscles can push you for running. Since you cannot push back at the ground while you are pushing forward to lift, gravity is the only force that can push you forward. To make gravity pull you harder, change your balance by dropping your feet back closer to an upright standing position.

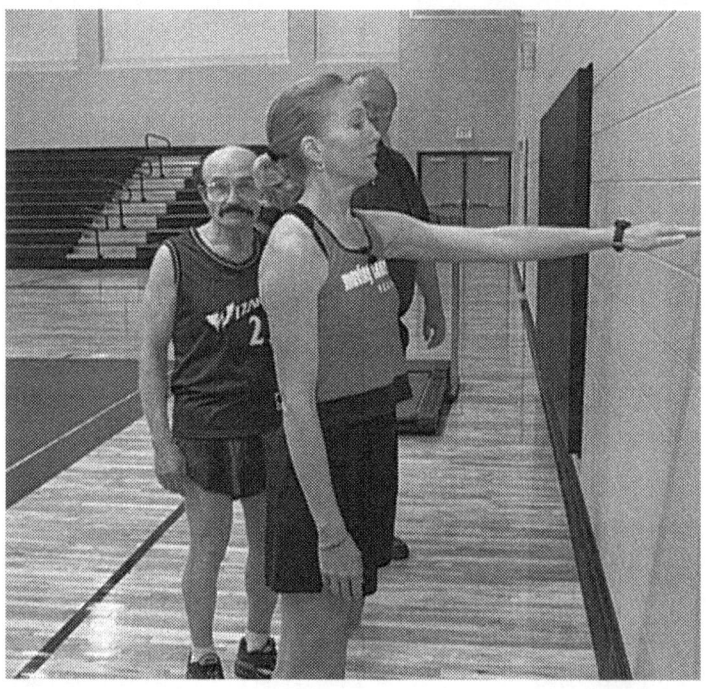

Professionals can't admit to the fact that your muscles can't push your body forward. For one thing, it's the basis for their techniques. Another thing is that they might not be able to grasp my gravity technique enough to qualify them as a real expert. Take the test pictured above and see if it easy for you to understand it. Touch the wall with your fingers and step back a little so that your weight, being pulled by gravity, is pressing your fingertips. Push your feet back with your leg muscles to add more pressure against your fingertips. You will be surprised that you can't add any more pressure to your fingertips. Your muscles are pushing the ground forward to support you and won't drop that support to let you push back. Only gravity is available as an option to push you forward.

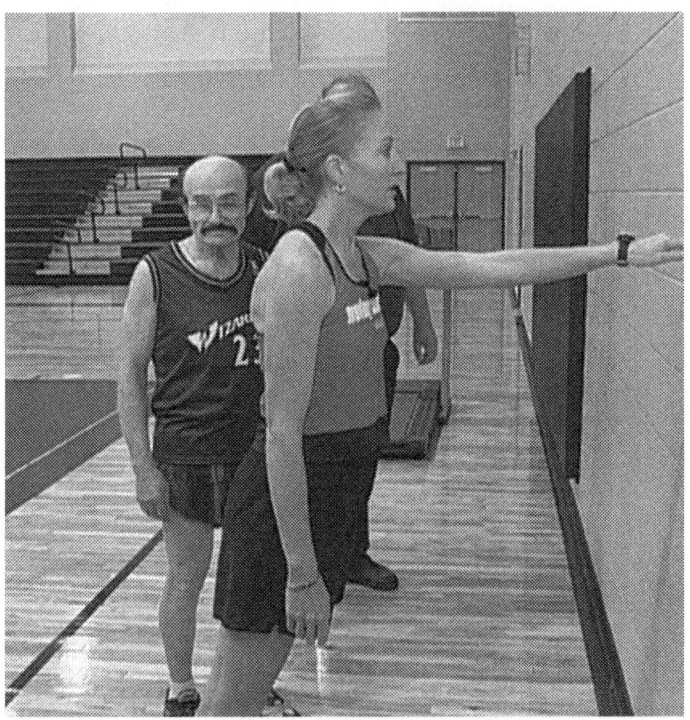

Step back further from the wall and feel the greater pressure against your fingertips. With your weight far ahead of your feet, gravity pulls you much harder. Push back with your muscles and notice that you cannot add pressure to your fingertips, no matter how hard you push. Now do something that will surprise you even more: Jump forward and notice that you still can't add pressure to your fingertips. The jump can only take you straight up. The fall while jumping is how you jump forward. Because you didn't increase your weight shift, the jump didn't make you go forward.

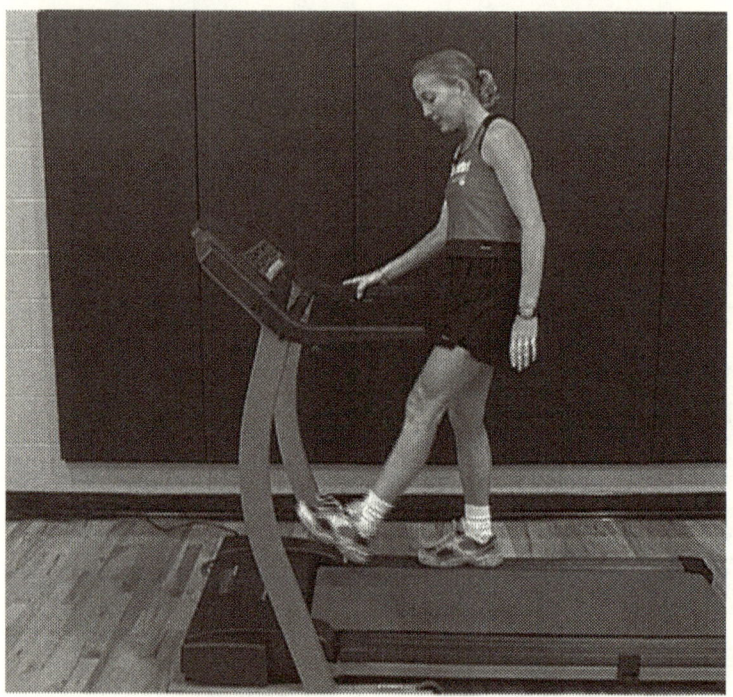

Overstriding and then dropping the foot down and back before it hits the ground is what many runners do, especially elite runners. They do not do it properly, though. Their objective is to push back at the ground faster than it is moving away. They are under the false impression that they can hit back against the ground to push themselves forward. Because all you are able to actually do is stand without pushing back and let gravity roll your foot forward, all runners traumatize their hamstrings muscles, many times stressing the hamstrings to the point of tearing them. This dangerous method is popularized by what is called the "pawback" method. It is the current standard that my technique proves to be wrong.

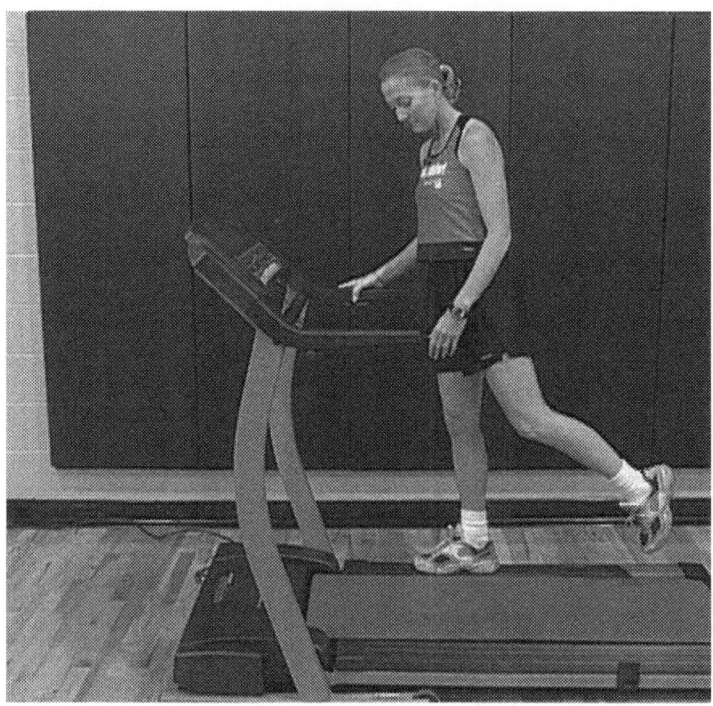

Stand on the frame of the treadmill next to a slow-moving belt and try the overstride technique using the right way. Bring your foot forward over the moving belt. Now let it drop down and back. The backward action should match the speed of the belt. Immediately after touching down, stand neutral without pushing back at the ground. Feel the ground pulling the foot back as if you are standing still on a moving platform. When the foot leaves the ground, do not lift it back and up; the foot will flip back by the momentum from the speed at which it was going on the belt. Bringing the foot back wastes time and energy in the process of exchanging the feet. A slow-moving belt, which is in effect a slow running pace, will not flip the leg back far and high up.

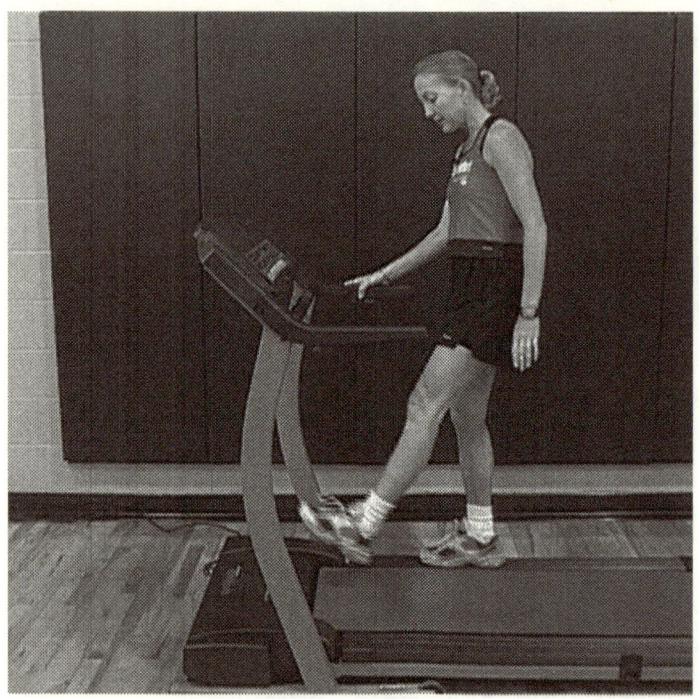

The toe should be kept up as it sweeps forward along the ground to prevent you from tripping. As the foot drops back and down, the toe should be lowered to a point slightly higher than the heel. This will allow you to touch the ground lightly with the flat part of the heel. When the weight comes down, the foot should be flat to absorb the pressure over a wide area of the foot. Since you are touching down by lowering the foot while in suspended animation, there is no severe impact on landing. Shown above, the foot is about to be lowered on to a speeding belt. You need to keep that in mind when running on a treadmill: The ground (treadmill belt) is always moving away from you fast when you are running fast. Hitting against the ground is high impact to your joints. The over-stride, then the dropping back and lowering of the foot while airborne, not only prevents injuries but also adds speed. An abrupt landing cuts speed.

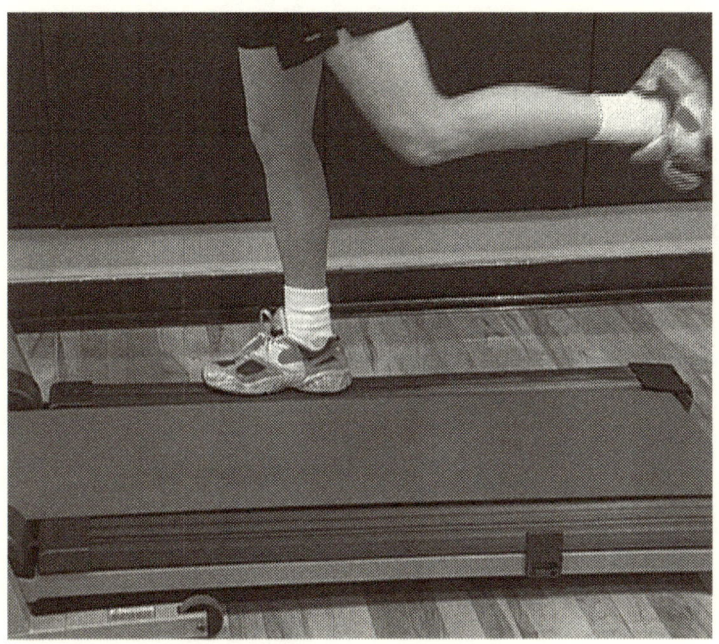

With a faster belt speed, the foot coming off of the belt has greater momentum, which swings it faster and farther back and up. All pushing power should be stopped a split second after touching down. You should feel the ground dragging your foot back the rest of the way and flipping the foot off the ground. You just stand while rolling forward on the foot, as you do when standing still. Gravity will roll you forward on your ankle and foot. The foot takes a longer swing back after it leaves the ground and has a longer distance to return to the front for a landing. As a result, you cannot exchange the feet as quickly at a fast pace as you can at a slow pace. At a fast pace your legs are returned with faster swings but the longer distance takes more time.

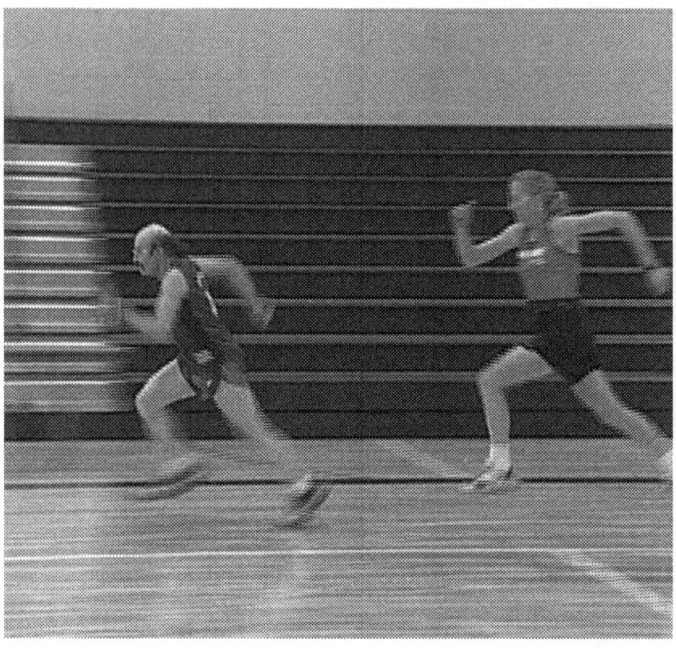

The two runners are racing each other while testing the standard technique against my technique, the Nirenstein technique. The runner in front is using the power of gravity more efficiently than the runner behind. The second runner is using the poor but standard technique of pushing off of the toes too hard, which makes you jump too high. The knee is raised too high, which wastes time in returning the foot to the ground. The higher jump makes for a longer stride that is part of the slowdown phase of the stride cycle. Gravity slows you when your foot is not on the ground behind your body. The air time and the first part of the support time (landing) are the slowdown phase. Using your power to lengthen the stride instead of using your power to shorten it slows you. Dropping the feet more to the rear gets a harder push from gravity. The schooled runners who run contrary to what they are taught are the ones that become champions. Their coaches take the undeserved credit.

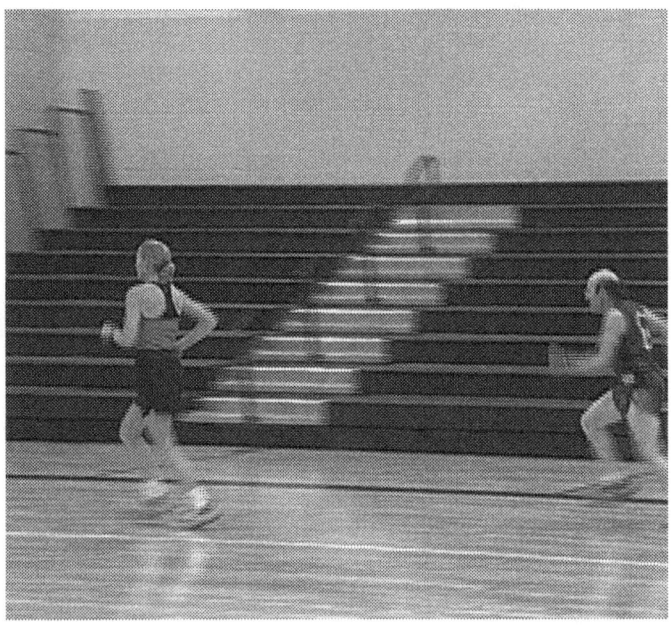

The runners switched techniques. The runner in front is now using the Nirenstein technique. The runner behind is using the standard way. The runner in front is using power to keep the stride from spreading apart. It can't be prevented from spreading, but it can be contained to a shorter spread. The foot is being pushed forward along with the knee. The knee stays low to keep the foot low, in order to help in a faster exchange of the feet. There is no pushing back at the ground. The leg is just used for support while it is being pulled back by the ground. A body twist from the upper arms and shoulders to the feet makes for more power to drive the foot forward. It was easy for the front runner to switch her style to a more efficient way. When you know that gravity is the forward motion force, it is easy to make yourself fall faster forward. A new group of coaches needs to be teaching the Nirenstein technique to make running a safer and easier sport.

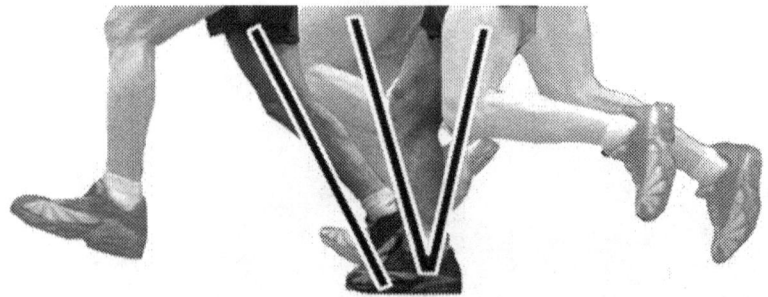

A key factor that led to the confusion of running experts is that they didn't take note of the way the legs act like a vaulting pole. Most people have seen pictures of runners with their foot on the ground ahead of their body. They also have seen pictures of the same runners with their foot far behind. The experts never noticed that the foot stays on the ground motionless while the hip never stops. When the foot is on the ground, the leg takes the photo position you've seen in which the foot is in front of the body. The foot stays still while the leg swings forward to the position you've seen in the other photo with the foot behind the body. A vaulting pole doing a horizontal vault follows the same motion. In running, the legs are locked at the hinges (joints) and swing around the foot. As it swings forward the leg rolls on the foot.

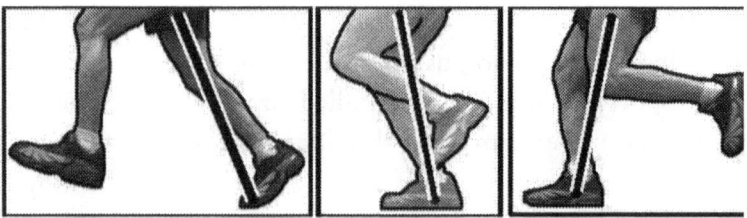

Starting from right to left, the first clip shows the first stage of the vaulting process during the support phase of the stride in a run. The foot has landed ahead of the body. Momentum is pushing the hip forward while the foot is motionless on the ground. The second clip shows the foot in the same place as it is in the first clip. The hip has moved forward and is now ahead of the foot. The leg is rolling forward on the ankle, in the socket of the foot. Momentum has carried the hip forward and the leg has vaulted the hip ahead of the foot. The third clip shows the foot in the same place on the ground as it is in the two previous clips. The hip has fallen forward and down while it was being pulled by gravity. The leg has been extended by the rotation of the knee and ankle joints to send the hip up and glide level with the ground. Now the leg is continuing to roll forward on the toe. The support phase in the stride has a slowdown phase (clip 1) in which the foot is ahead of the body and working against gravity. Then comes a pickup phase, during which the body passes the foot (clips 2 and 3). The leg is falling and extending while it is being pulled by gravity. The balanced slowdown and pickup phases keep you at an even pace. Reaching six inches ahead of the body for a landing gives you a slower pace than landing five inches ahead.

My basic discovery is that everyone runs the same way without knowing what it is. If you are not falling forward, you cannot be moving forward to walk or run. The pull of gravity will not let you stand still when your foot/feet are not centered under your body. You cannot jump from one spot to another unless you fall first then lift as you are falling. No pushing back at the ground can push you forward, or you would run faster on the moon than you can on earth.

978-0-595-40757-6
0-595-40757-9